the**facts**

Falls

➔ also available in the**facts** series

the**facts**

Falls

DR ADAM DAROWSKI MD FRCP

Consultant Physician
Nuffield Department of Medicine
John Radcliffe Hospital
Oxford

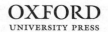
OXFORD
UNIVERSITY PRESS

OXFORD
UNIVERSITY PRESS

Great Clarendon Street, Oxford OX2 6DP

Oxford University Press is a department of the University of Oxford.
It furthers the University's objective of excellence in research, scholarship,
and education by publishing worldwide in

Oxford New York

Auckland Cape Town Dar es Salaam Hong Kong Karachi
Kuala Lumpur Madrid Melbourne Mexico City Nairobi
New Delhi Shanghai Taipei Toronto

With offices in

Argentina Austria Brazil Chile Czech Republic France Greece
Guatemala Hungary Italy Japan Poland Portugal Singapore
South Korea Switzerland Thailand Turkey Ukraine Vietnam

Oxford is a registered trade mark of Oxford University Press
in the UK and in certain other countries

Published in the United States
by Oxford University Press Inc., New York

British Library Cataloguing in Publication Data

Data available

Library of Congress Cataloging in Publication Data
Darowski, Adam.
 Falls: the facts / Adam Darowski.
  p. cm. — (The facts)
 Includes index.
 ISBN-13: 978-0-19-954128-7
 1. Falls (Accidents) I. Title.
 RD93.D37 2008
 613.6—dc22

                                                                    2008005964

ISBN 978-0-19-954128-7

10 9 8 7 6 5 4 3 2 1

Typeset in Plantin
by Cepha Imaging Pvt. Ltd., Bangalore, India
Printed in China
through Asia Pacific Offset

Whilst every effort has been made to ensure that the contents of this book are as complete,
accurate, and up-to-date as possible at the date of writing, Oxford University Press is not able
to give any guarantee or assurance that such is the case. Readers are urged to take appropriately
qualified medical advice in all cases. The information in this book is intended to be useful to
the general reader, but should not be used as a means of self-diagnosis or for the prescription of
medication.

Foreword

Independence and a healthy active later life is a vision which many of us share and hope to achieve. But this requires a well-informed population; one that is aware of the increasing risk of falling as age increases as well as in receipt of the information and understanding of how to reduce or avoid falling altogether.

That is why this book is to be welcomed. It provides concise, helpful, and practical information for the lay person or their carer on the reasons why we tend to fall as we age and how the risk of falling can be reduced. With over two thousand people dying each year as a result of falling and others losing confidence and becoming isolated because of the fear of falling again, this book is timely.

There is always going to be a role for doctors, nurses, and other health practitioners in supporting us as we age. But reducing the risk of falling cannot be achieved without the individual taking some responsibility. It means making changes and modifications to the way we live and taking care to remain as fit and balanced as possible. With knowledge and understanding, this is achievable.

We at Help the Aged are passionate about a future where older people are physically and mentally fit, and we work hard to ensure the best possible quality of life for all of us as we age. This book plays its part in achieving our aim.

Pamela Holmes
Help the Aged

Preface

This book arose from the need to provide material for the training of nurses and therapists in the management of falls, and to have easily understood material available for our patients.

I have written a personal view of the subject as I see it, having run a falls clinic for 15 years. Research into falls is in its infancy. Where there is research evidence available, I have taken it into account, but there are large areas of the subject in which research is meagre. In particular, this applies to some of the problems arising from the heart and circulation, their diagnosis, and their treatments, and to the effects of medications. No doubt future research will clarify these areas.

Acknowledgements

I would like to apologize to my wife and children for the large amount of family time they have foregone to allow me to write this book, and to thank them for their patience. Many people have helped me along the way, in particular the staff of the Oxfordshire Falls Service and the Lionel Cosin Day Hospital. The book would never have seen the light of day without the encouragement of Antoinette Broad. My thanks go to all of those who have read and commented on various parts of the book while it was in preparation, in particular Kris Silvester, Trish Astle, Esther Bayer, Louise Spoors, Jenny Watson, Anne-Marie Probert, and Sheena Davie. I would like to thank those who have read the book when finished to see if it made sense—David Oliver, Finbarr Martin, Ian Philp, Sallie Lamb, and Maura Buchanan.

Contents

1

Introduction

 Key points

Falls are common.

Falls can be serious because they cause injuries.

Something can always be done to diminish the chances of further falls or to make the environment safer.

Falls can be divided into several groups:

- accidents, trips and slips

- falls due to an illness causing weakness or unsteadiness

- falls due to an innate tendency to fall

- falls due to faintness or loss of consciousness.

Commonly, any given individual will fall into more than one of these categories, and usually there are multiple causes for falls.

Falls are common

We all fall occasionally, but as people grow older they fall more frequently, and they start to fall at moments when they would not have expected to. After the age of 65, about a third of people fall every year, and after the age of 80 this

1

proportion rises to a half. Most people fall at some stage, but if falls recur they should not just be dismissed as part of growing old.

- ◆ Falls can be simple accidents—trips and slips. These account for most falls.

- ◆ Some people who are otherwise fit and well fall down with no obvious explanation. Such unexplained falls often have an underlying cause. Many of these falls are associated with problems with the heart or circulation, or a brief period of loss of consciousness.

- ◆ Recurrent falls happen to those who have some deterioration in their gait or balance, or some pre-existing illness or disability.

These groups of falls blend together—people who have poor balance can slip, and their stumble is more likely to result in a fall. Those who already suffer from recurrent falls are just as likely as anyone else to have other falls due to changes in their pulse or blood pressure.

Very often patients will rationalize their falls, and say that they had an accident when there is some other underlying cause. In such cases the doctor may be dissuaded from taking matters further, and significant treatable problems may be missed.

Once someone has had two or more falls that have no clear explanation, it is likely that they will have further falls and they ought to seek medical attention.

Falls can be serious

Sportsmen fall over all the time, and for them it is generally no more harmful than sneezing. Older people are frailer and have thinner bones. Their protective

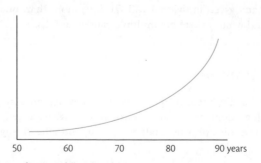

Figure 1.1 Rate of serious falls-related injury versus age.

responses are less effective. They are more prone to injury. It is the injuries that make falls so important.

Falls are preventable in many cases

For anyone who has falls, things can be done to diminish the chances of further falls or to reduce the risk of injury if there is a fall. There are many things that increase the risk of falls, and the more risk factors someone has the greater is their risk of falling. Not all of these factors can be removed, but it is important to minimize those that can be changed.

2

How do we stay upright?

→ Key points

Sensations concerning position and movement are sent to the brain from:

- nerves providing body sensation
- the eyes
- the inner ear.

The brain interprets these, and decides what responses are needed.

Instructions in the form of nerve impulses are sent to muscles around the body to make the movements that the brain thinks are necessary.

Movements are made by muscles in specific areas, with certain muscle groups acting together in such a way as to maintain or restore balance. These movements and adjustments are very rapid, and are largely subconscious.

Any discussion of why we fall must start with an understanding of how we manage to stay upright. A large part of the nervous system is involved in maintaining balance, and the following account is very simplified.

The system that maintains balance needs to be very quick and accurate if we are to withstand the threats to our balance posed by normal activities such as walking, let alone unexpected things such as trips or being pushed. Most of the control of balance is subconscious.

Balance control

Controlling balance can be considered in two parts, one concerned with recognizing position in space, and the other with restoring the body to a balanced position. This involves many decisions to perform movements, often made consciously to carry out a specific task. These are accompanied by numerous other balancing movements which the body makes subconsciously. With age, the subconscious part becomes less reliable, slower, and less accurate, and more conscious thought is required to maintain balance.

Being 'in balance' means that the centre of gravity is kept within an area above our feet known as the 'base of support'. This is the area above which we are stable. Once the centre of gravity moves outside the base of support, we need to make a movement to change our position, or else we will fall over. We expend the smallest amount of energy when we are standing vertically above our base of support, and this is the easiest position for the body to maintain.

The brain has developed so as to be very sensitive in detecting where the vertical lies. This is fundamental to maintaining balance. A normal person standing in the dark can recognize a movement away from the vertical of as little as a half a degree.

> A distinction needs to be made between the demands of standing, called **static balance**, and those of movement, called **dynamic balance**.
>
> **Dynamic balance** demands thought, judgement, and anticipation. Moving the body causes us to put ourselves off balance temporarily, having planned how we will regain balance with another movement.

Sensations from nerves around the body, from the eyes, and from the organ of balance in the inner ear tell the brain where the body is in space.

Body sensation (proprioception)

There is a system of nerves coming from all the muscles, joints, and tendons in the body carrying information to the brain about movement and position. Other nerves provide information about how strongly our muscles are contracting. These provide the main sensations that tell us where we are in space.

In addition, we receive information from nerves telling us about skin sensations. When sitting in an armchair, a large part of the body is in contact with the chair, giving rise to sensory information for the brain to work on. On standing, only the soles of the feet are in contact with a firm surface.

The deterioration in body sensation with age is thought to be one of the most important factors leading to the increase in the tendency to fall with increasing age.

📄 Case history

David was a 78-year-old man who had his right leg amputated above the knee in his thirties following an accident. He had a prosthesis fitted, and worked normally until retirement.

He had several admissions with falls. Three years previously he had a left hip replacement. He had normally made more use of his left leg to stand on, so as not to put weight through his stump, leading to an increased burden on the left hip joint which eventually led to arthritis.

He said that when he first lost his leg and got his new prosthesis he could feel what was under his right shoe almost normally—if he stood on a matchstick he would be aware of it. Now he had much less sensation through the stump.

The disease and eventual replacement of his hip meant that he had lost some of the sensory input from his previously good leg. He had now reached a stage where he was not receiving enough sensory information from his legs to keep himself balanced.

He accepted the need to walk with sticks, and after some training regained his confidence and independence.

We all do things that give us helpful additional body sensations. Touching a piece of furniture as we cross the room, running the back of a hand along a wall when walking down a corridor, and using a stick to tell where the floor is (rather than for support) are all important practical things that demonstrate the importance of body sensation.

Vestibular sensation

The organ of balance in the inner ear consists of three canals arranged in semi-circles, each at right angles to the others (Figure 2.1). Movement of the head causes movement of fluid within the semicircular canals, and this is detected by hair cells at one end of each canal. Each canal gives information about movement in that plane, and the existence of three canals means that a judgement can be made about movements in any direction.

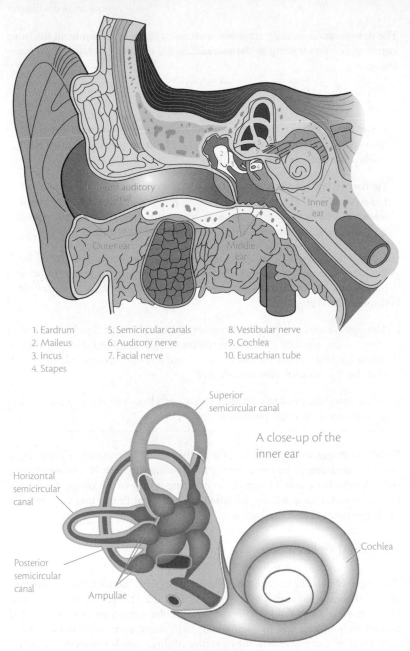

1. Eardrum
2. Maileus
3. Incus
4. Stapes
5. Semicircular canals
6. Auditory nerve
7. Facial nerve
8. Vestibular nerve
9. Cochlea
10. Eustachian tube

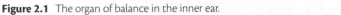

Figure 2.1 The organ of balance in the inner ear.

If the vestibular apparatus is damaged, it creates a sensation of imbalance that is difficult to correct. Typically, there is a sensation of instability or vertigo (a sensation of movement, usually spinning, without any real movement occurring).

Vision

Visual function can be affected in several different ways.

◆ **Visual acuity** is the term used to describe our ability to see things clearly, either in the distance or when reading. Acuity is impaired when the lens in the eye lets light through, but does not focus it accurately on the retina at the back of the eye. If the lens is normal, this aspect of poor vision can be corrected by simple spectacles.

◆ **Double vision** occurs when the eyes point in slightly different directions. Anything that affects the nerves supplying the eye muscles, those parts of the brain controlling eye muscles, or, less commonly, the muscles themselves will result in double vision.

◆ **Depth perception** is the ability to decide the distances between things that are in front of you. **Stereoscopic vision**, the use of information from both eyes to judge distance, plays some part in this. However, we are still able to judge distance with one eye closed, or look at a picture and assess depth. One important aspect of visual perception is the 'wallpaper illusion'. When looking at a repetitive horizontal pattern, each eye may fix upon a different part of the pattern, leading to confused visual inputs. This is even more important when the horizontal lines are moving—for example, as at the top of an escalator looking at the steps moving downwards. This creates a misunderstanding of position, and has been shown to cause falls on escalators.

◆ **Contrast sensitivity** is the ability to see where one thing finishes and another starts. For example, when walking down a flight of stairs in poor lighting, it may be difficult to tell where one step finishes and the next begins.

Integration of information in the brain

Sensory information feeds into the brain, which then has to put it all together to work out where the body is in space and then carry out appropriate movements to maintain or restore balance.

◆ **Sensory nerves** feed into the spinal cord (Figure 2.2), which enters the bottom part of the brain—the brainstem.

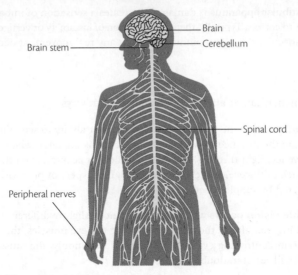

Brain
Cerebellum
Brain stem
Spinal cord
Peripheral nerves

Figure 2.2 The nervous system.

◆ At the back of the brainstem lies the **cerebellum**, a part of the brain almost entirely devoted to the control of balance, integrating sensory information about position and initiating automatic movements to maintain balance.

◆ **Information from the vestibular system** enters the brainstem and makes an abundant network of connections to various parts of the brain.

Conscious decisions about movement are made in the higher parts of the brain, and those instructions are sent down to the muscles through the cerebellum and brainstem.

◆ **Information from the eyes** goes through the brain from front to back—a long connection that leaves it very vulnerable to damage in various parts of the brain. It is then put together in the back of the brain, and this information is shared through connections with those parts of the brain concerned with balance.

The limits of stability

Above our base of support is an imaginary inverted cone, which represents the area within which we can move our body without losing balance. This is termed the limit of stability (Figure 2.3). Any movement that takes the centre

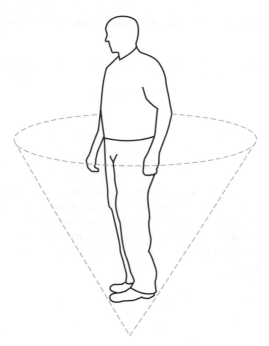

Figure 2.3 The limits of stability.

of gravity outside the limits of stability leads to an automatic movement to reposition the body and restore balance. If that corrective movement is not made, balance is lost, and the result is a fall.

- ❖ **Postural responses** may be anticipatory or reactive.

- ❖ **Anticipatory responses** occur when movements or changes in balance are planned in advance. This happens every time you take a step. As you lift up one leg, your weight moves forward onto the ball of the foot that is still on the ground, and you are in an unstable position until your other foot hits the ground, restoring your base of support.

- ❖ **Reactive responses** occur when unexpected forces act on the body and disturb balance. An example is when a bus moves off suddenly with you standing up inside it. Your feet are on the floor of the bus, and will move with respect to your body, which will feel as though it has jerked back-wards. You will make an automatic movement with your feet to move them backwards, so that your body once again comes to be in a position above your feet.

Whereas a younger person would anticipate these changes and make the necessary adjustments without thinking about them, with increasing age the automatic part of the response is less reliable, and more thought is required to make the right movements.

Responses occur too quickly for them to be voluntary movements, and they are generated by those parts of the brain that respond automatically—primarily the cerebellum. These automatic responses are slowed by ageing.

Anticipation of having to make movements to correct the imbalance that is expected following any movement is a vital part of the process of remaining upright. It is one of the key things a toddler has to master in order to walk unaided, and one of those things that becomes impaired in some older people. It is a subconscious awareness of position that produces semi-automatic corrective movements.

3

Why do people fall?

➡ Key points

The chances of falling increase with:

- increasing age

- medications that affect balance and alertness

- increasing sensory loss—vision, body sensation, vestibular sensation

- disability

- diseases, particularly stroke and Parkinson's disease

- memory loss and dementia.

35 per cent of people over 65 years old and 50 per cent of those over 80 fall each year.

Falls are usually due to more than one factor.

There is commonly a combination of:

- **intrinsic factors**—a susceptibility to falling

- **extrinsic factors**—situations or events in which balance is challenged.

Dogs rarely fall. A dog has a leg at each corner and a low centre of gravity. It takes considerable effort to push a dog over. It is intrinsically stable.

People have a high centre of gravity; they have to balance on two legs, and maintaining stability is much more difficult. During the process of evolution from a four-legged to a two-legged animal, we have had to develop a complex system that enables us to balance and to walk on two legs.

This system has to be robust enough to withstand a variety of threats to balance. Not falling in response to such a threat depends upon knowing where the body is in space, understanding how its balance has been perturbed, and then making the right responses to restore balance in time to prevent a fall.

Of the three types of sensation reaching the brain, body sensation (proprioception) seems to be the most important in maintaining balance. Balance can usually be maintained if vision is lost or the inner ear is damaged, as long as proprioception remains intact.

❓ Why do older people fall over more often?

Older people fall because the balance system as a whole is less sensitive, less rapid, less accurate, and weaker.

There are numerous causes. Diminished sensory input is a major factor. Degeneration of the nerves of body sensation with age or illness has been considered the main problem, but the degeneration of connections within the brain (cerebral small vessel disease) may be more important. In addition, those parts that carry out the movements (muscles and joints) may be weak, damaged, or painful.

Many factors can affect the brain's ability to process sensory information properly. In older people, the most common, and possibly the most important, is small vessel disease affecting the brain (see Chapter 13). This poorly understood condition is so common as to be almost normal with increasing age. Deeper areas of the brain have some damage to their blood supply, leading to small areas of cell death and disruption to pathways carrying impulses from one part of the brain to another. Some authorities consider this to be the main reason for the increase in falls with age.

Other neurological diseases, such as Parkinson's disease and stroke contribute to an increased risk of falls through a variety of effects (see Chapter 13).

An example of impaired processing of information by the brain often seen in younger people is too much alcohol. While excessive drinking is probably less common in older people, they are much more likely to be taking medications that will affect balance, such as sleeping tablets and antidepressants. The effect is very similar.

Commonly, older people also take medications that affect the blood supply to the brain by causing a reduction in blood pressure. Their reduced reserves make them more susceptible than the young to the side effects of medicines.

Even when the brain is supplied with good quality sensory information and is functioning normally, so that this information is processed correctly, there may still be reasons why someone may have a tendency to fall. If the muscles are weak, or if they have to work around joints that are painful because of arthritis, or if there is damage to the nerves that send impulses down the muscles, there will be some impairment of balance and an increased likelihood of falling.

Not concentrating on balance can also lead to falls. This may be simple carelessness, but anxiety, depression, or confusion may prevent someone from concentrating sufficiently on what they are doing. Occasionally, patients simply seem unconcerned by the need to focus on where they are placing their feet, and fall as a result.

There are numerous other factors which may come into play that can make someone less able to withstand threats to their balance. These may be simple things such as an infection, or any other illness that makes the patient feel unwell. It is well recognized that falling can be a manifestation of any illness in an older person. Disability from other illnesses may also affect balance.

Causes of falls are divided into two groups.

Intrinsic factors are things to do with the person: a bad knee that gives way, an illness, a previous stroke, side effects of medication, etc.

Extrinsic factors are those in the environment: something to trip over, a slippery floor, being pushed, the bus moving off suddenly, etc.

As we grow older, all the mechanisms for maintaining balance work less well. As a result the rate of falling increases with increasing age. Research has shown that about 35 per cent of people over the age of 65 fall each year, and for people over the age of 80 the chance of a fall is 50 per cent in any given year.

With additional problems, the chances of falling rise further still. Studies have shown that people with Parkinson's disease have a 38–53 per cent chance of falling in a year. Frail older people are two or three times more likely to fall than those who are vigorous. Those who have already had a fall are much more likely to have further falls: 57 per cent will have a fall in the year after their first fall, and 31 per cent will have two or more falls.

There are several well-recognized circumstances associated with falling.

◆ Collisions in the dark, usually on getting out of bed at night, are one of the most common.

◆ Forgetting about temporary hazards around the home—something left out of place, or something new that they are not used to.

◆ Slipping or catching a toe on a carpet is very common,

◆ Simple carelessness about the house.

There is usually a mixture of extrinsic factors such as these, which combine with things that cause an intrinsic tendency to have falls, such as impaired vision, poor balance, giddiness, or the effects of medicines.

People who manage to live on their own at home are less likely to fall than those who live in retirement communities. Those who live in residential homes are at the highest risk of falling. In part, this is because recurrent falls are one of the main reasons why people give up living alone at home and move into a care home. Their risk of falling is especially high in the first few weeks when their new surroundings are unfamiliar.

Once patients are no longer able to walk or stand, their risk of falling naturally reduces, but they may continue to have falls while attempting to transfer from bed or chair to the toilet, and may fall out of bed.

4

What causes simple falls? Trips, slips, and the effects of illness

> ### → Key points
>
> ◆ About half of falls are simple falls due to a slip or a trip.
>
> ◆ Short-term illnesses commonly result in falls.
>
> ◆ A fall associated with giddiness, loss of consciousness, or awareness of an abnormal heart beat needs further evaluation by a doctor.

Trips and slips

Most falls are due to simple trips and slips of the sort that we all experience from time to time. Most older people who fall do not need any specialist intervention. Most do not ever see a doctor or nurse and find that they have soon forgotten all about it.

The problem arises when the falls start to recur and to form a pattern. Those aspects of ageing discussed elsewhere start to play a role. Impaired vision and loss of sensory input from the inner ear and from peripheral nerves, together with a slowing of reaction times, all play a part in turning a stumble into a fall. Other illnesses or disabilities which might have been present for years— the arthritic knee, the mild Parkinson's disease, the old stroke, the peripheral neuropathy—now contribute to impaired walking or balance in a way that they did not before.

Commonly, people say that they tripped up on the kerb or on a loose paving stone. What needs to be explained is why they have tripped twice on a paving stone in the last few weeks, but have never done so for the preceding 80 years of their lives. There is usually some underlying cause for this sort of repeated event. People who go down without really understanding why they fell, and those who feel that they may have passed out usually have a significant underlying medical problem, and need further evaluation by their doctor.

Illness

Falling is one of the most common reasons for an older person to be admitted to hospital. For most, this is their first or only fall, and they have fallen as a result of their illness rather than from any native tendency to fall.

Almost any illness in an older person can result in fall, often termed 'a collapse' when they arrive in hospital. The most common reasons are infections and the side effects of medications (see Chapter 10). Fever has an effect on the brain, and makes even young people unsteady on their feet. In older people it commonly leads to dehydration and may cause confusion. It exaggerates the side effects of medications.

Deranged metabolism, in the form of a low blood sugar, kidney failure, or low levels of sodium or potassium in the blood, can all contribute to falls

Many heart conditions can lead to a sudden collapse. These include heart attacks, irregular heart rhythms, and clots in the lungs. Any condition that causes localized weakness or sudden pain will cause people to fall.

These cases differ from those described elsewhere in this book. While those with an inherent tendency to fall are much more likely to do so when they are ill, most of these patients do not have a tendency to fall, and once their underlying problem has been dealt with they do not fall again.

Seeking medical attention

When should someone who has had a fall seek specialist advice? Many people who have never fallen seek advice because they feel unsteady and fear that they might fall. Some people who fall continually do not want any advice. In general, however, there are certain recognized levels at which help should be sought.

You should seek medical attention if:

- you have had two or more falls in the last year that cannot be explained

- you have had a single fall associated with loss of consciousness, giddi-ness, or a rapid or forceful heart beat

- you have had a single fall that has caused significant injury

- you have fear of further falling

- you were unable to get up off the floor when you fell.

In addition, many patients are referred who have frequent or persistent giddiness and unsteadiness, as the causes for these are often the same as those for falls.

5

How do poor balance and muscle weakness contribute to falls?

→ **Key points**

◆ A large proportion of all falls occur because of the combination of impaired balance and weak muscles.

◆ Both of these factors become common with increasing age, and usually both are present when someone who has fallen is seen in the clinic.

◆ Trying to work out which is the major factor in any individual is often impossible, as they are inextricably linked.

Muscle weakness

Muscle weakness has many causes:

◆ any illness will cause muscle weakness

◆ painful joints cause loss of muscle around the joint, with weakness and a tendency for the joint to give way

◆ previous injury, surgery, or disability, especially in the legs

◆ prolonged immobility causes wasting and weakness

◆ deconditioning—not using the muscles enough—is very common

◆ specific neurological conditions such as stroke and neuropathy lead to weakness

◆ poor nutrition, especially vitamin D deficiency, causes muscle wasting

◆ prolonged use of steroid tablets

◆ hormonal problems—thyroid disease, low testosterone levels.

As people grow older the nervous system and the muscles degenerate. Muscle bulk is lost. It is difficult to determine how much of this is due simply to doing less, and how much is due to the ageing process or illness.

In some people the effect of long-standing poor nutrition plays a part, and in others muscle lost during an illness is never replaced during convalescence.

Muscle weakness is often associated with illness. Any sort of severe illness makes us feel weak; a prolonged period in bed makes things much worse.

📄 Case history

Ethel was an 86-year-old woman admitted following a fall at home. She was almost completely deaf, and communication was by her response to written questions.

She had obviously lost weight, but on the ward appeared to be hungry and to have a good appetite. She had injured her hip and could not walk. There was no fracture, and over a couple of weeks she regained her mobility.

About a week after admission, the nurses noted that she regurgitated some of her food after each meal, something she had felt embarrassed about and had tried to hide from the nurses.

An endoscopy was done to examine her stomach, and this found a tight narrowing at the lower end of the oesophagus—a benign oesophageal stricture. This was dilated (a simple procedure taking a few minutes done under sedation) and subsequently she was able to swallow normally.

She then ate normally, put on weight, and gained strength. She had no further falls, and after a period of weeks went back to her own home, walking well, and able to look after herself.

She had fallen because of the muscular weakness caused by her weight loss. She had lost weight because of her oesophageal stricture.

Older people do not have the same reserves and are likely to be affected more severely. It may take many weeks for them to regain their strength.

In addition, many people are affected by conditions that make their muscles weaker. Arthritis is probably the most common of these. If there is a painful or diseased joint, there is loss of the muscle around the joint. It is not uncommon for people to have arthritis affecting both knees and both hips. This will contribute to falling not only because of the weakness, but also because of the tendency of painful joints to give way, and because painful joints change the way we walk to one that is less secure.

Stroke is the most common neurological condition leading to muscle weakness. People can have small vessel disease or have numerous small strokes without being aware of it, and these have a cumulative effect on the brain and on muscle strength.

The effects of muscle weakness on balance

Generalized muscular weakness leads to a sensation of imbalance. If the muscles are weak, the ability to make corrective movements to restore balance will be affected. The muscles may not be able to generate enough power to make the movements needed to prevent a fall, particularly when faced with a sudden threat to balance while walking, when a stumble is more likely to result in a fall.

Weakness affects posture, which can leave the body in an unbalanced position. For example, someone with a painful knee may put all their weight on their good leg to protect the painful joint. They will stand in a way that leaves them more vulnerable to any threat to their balance.

Weakness affects the way we walk, and walking is likely to be less safe, as the muscle groups needed to restore balance at every step will not be strong enough to do their job properly.

Case history

Anna was a 62-year-old woman with a long history of falls, but with several falls in recent months. She had congenital dislocation of the hip as a child, which had not been treated, leaving her with painful hip joints and a waddling gait. At the age of 16 her right hip had been fused to the pelvis. As a result the muscles of her thigh and buttock had almost vanished.

She had a history of vertigo 10 years previously, for which no clear diagnosis had been established. It had resolved, but left her with impaired balance.

Five years previously, at the age of 57, she had an operation on the fused hip and a total hip replacement. Her falls had become worse at about this time.

She was unable to stand with her feet together, starting to fall to the right within a couple of seconds. The muscles of her buttock on the right, which maintain sideways stability, were almost absent, and she was unable to hold herself up at the right hip joint. The whole of the right leg was weak, and she could not generate the power in her leg to make adequate corrective movements. Her sense of falling was impaired by her long-standing inner ear problems.

For 40 years she had not had to use her buttock muscles to stabilize her hip joint, as it had been fused to her pelvis. When the hip joint was replaced, she did not have the muscle strength to keep it stable, and started to fall. Once the problem had been diagnosed, she started exercises to strengthen the muscles around her hip and used a stick to improve her stability.

The impairment of sensory inputs to balance

Sensory inputs to balance can be impaired with ageing and disease:

- nerves of body sensation deteriorate

- balance information from the inner ear deteriorates

- vision can be impaired by having the wrong glasses, or by diseases of the eye or the brain.

The balance problems that develop with age have many contributory factors, and each of the inputs to the balance system can be affected by ageing or disease.

Body sensation and ageing

Proprioception deteriorates with age in most people. It is very difficult to measure proprioception directly, as it is an awareness of movement and position, and is a subjective sensation.

The nerves that supply proprioception are closely related to those that supply vibration sense, which is much easier to measure (by assessing how long the buzzing of a tuning fork is felt). Vibration sense has long been known to be less sensitive with age. This deterioration in vibration sense is greater in the legs than in the arms, which is as expected because the nerves supplying the legs are longer and therefore more prone to damage or disease along their length. When groups of fallers are compared with non-fallers, they have significantly worse vibration sense and proprioception in the legs.

Vestibular information and ageing

Vestibular sensation has been found to be diminished with age in about a third of older people. The tests for vestibular function are very imprecise, and it is difficult to know if the abnormalities observed are significant. There is no doubt that some people with deranged vestibular function are unsteady, but little consistent relationship has been found between falls and vestibular function.

Those who have impaired vestibular function generally benefit from education about maintaining safety, and from walking aids when needed. In some cases exercises to accustom the brain to the abnormal information coming from a diseased inner ear can help the patient overcome the disability by making their brain more used to it.

Poor vision

Poor vision has been found to be a risk factor for falling in the elderly in a number of studies. The problem can lie at one or more levels. It may simply be one of getting the right glasses for eyes that are otherwise healthy. Alternatively, the eyes may be diseased, and visual information may be limited by the effects of that disease:

◆ in some cases the eye muscles do not work together, producing double vision

◆ following a stroke, or in other diseases affecting the brain, the brain may not interpret the visual information that it is receiving correctly.

Even in people with healthy eyes, vision can be poor because they need glasses. Bifocal glasses have two prescriptions—one for long sight and one for short sight—and may distort vision in the lower part of the lens, impairing the ability to judge the distance and height of steps or uneven surfaces. There is

25

evidence that both bifocals and varifocals increase the risk of falls compared with wearing glasses containing a single lens.

In situations in which visual information is ambiguous or poor, such as in poorly lit areas where the colours of surroundings are all similar, people may position their bodies wrongly based on inadequate visual information, and this may contribute to falls.

The brain's ability to interpret depth perception may be affected by diseases of the brain substance, such as stroke or Parkinson's disease. Any disease affecting the eyes, particularly those affecting the central part of vision (macular degeneration, cataract, or diabetes), will lead to less visual information reaching the brain, and greater difficulty in judging depth and distance.

Contrast sensitivity

For many older people seeing the edge of things such as stairs and kerbs is more difficult than for the young, and this may be a major cause of trips and slips, because it leads to errors in judgement as to where to place the feet.

The integration of sensory information in the brain

The integration of sensory inputs in the brain can be affected in many ways:

◆ stroke and small vessel disease of the brain interrupt pathways within the brain

◆ sleep loss, confusion, dementia, and illness will impair the way information is understood

◆ many medications will slow the working of the brain

◆ reaction times slow with age.

In the ageing brain there are commonly changes due to areas of inadequate blood supply. This is termed 'small vessel disease' or 'white matter change'. The result of this is that many areas of the brain work less well, leading to a general deterioration in all aspects of brain function. This is a major factor in many aspects of ageing, including deteriorating walking and balance.

These changes in the brain and peripheral nervous system affect our balance control. When we stand up, we do not stand perfectly still, but sway slightly backwards and forwards, and from side to side. As we grow older, we tend to sway more, and our stability limits become smaller. If our ability to obtain and interpret sensations is impaired, it becomes more likely that the stability limits will be exceeded. This leads to moments of imbalance, and an increased tendency to fall.

The awareness of vertical can be deranged with many conditions affecting the brain. When this occurs, a movement to restore the body to vertical may be done in error, and may lead to an unbalanced position, resulting in a fall.

Our ability to anticipate threats to our balance is also easily impaired. Anything that slows mental function will affect this. Any medicines that slow the working of the brain will affect our ability to plan our position ahead and make the appropriate anticipatory movements. Dementia, confusion, sleep loss, and illness will all increase the risk of falling by slowing or diminishing our ability to anticipate the movements we will need to make to maintain balance.

We can tell how well all of these mechanisms are working together by measuring reaction time. It tells us how rapidly the body responds to outside forces that challenge balance.

Reaction time can be measured in many ways, but that part related to balance is assessed by making the patient stand on a platform that can be moved suddenly from side to side (like standing in a bus that moves off suddenly). This platform is then moved suddenly a few centimetres to one side. The patient's feet will have been moved relative to the rest of the body, and the position of the feet and body will need to be readjusted. The speed with which such an adjustment is made can be measured, and gives us an idea of the patient's ability to react to a stimulus that puts them off balance.

Reaction times slow significantly with age. Response times increase by a quarter between the twenties and the sixties. Reaction times are strongly related to the risk of falls, because people do not respond quickly enough to reposition their bodies when put off balance. Many diseases affecting the brain, and many medicines, will slow reaction times.

It is not just the speed of the response that matters, but what the response consists of. The brain has to judge what the correct movement is to maintain balance, and carry it out at the right moment. It then has to have feedback from the body that balance has been restored, and has to interpret this correctly.

📄 Case history

Paul was an 80-year-old man who had difficulty walking, and had had several falls. These had started when on holiday he had suddenly felt a sharp pain in the back of his leg. This continued after his return home. He had suffered a tear of his right Achilles tendon, which had been left untreated and healed partially over a number of weeks. He was left with some weakness in his ability to lift his right foot—a partial foot drop.

He had been blind due to a hereditary condition affecting the optic nerves from his early twenties, and had spent his life working as a blind telephonist. In his forties he had been knocked down by a car, and had damaged his left leg badly, with a complex fracture of the lower leg and injury to the knee which required surgery. This had left him with a permanent moderate disability, and years later he had a left knee replacement. A few years after that he had a total right hip replacement.

He had a 30-year history of tablet-controlled diabetes, and had numbness in his feet from a diabetic peripheral neuropathy. About a year before coming to see me he had a stroke affecting his left arm, where he had persistent tingling and some mild weakness. There was also a story of several other mini-strokes over the years.

He had a number of factors contributing to his poor mobility and falls.

- He had a loss of sensory inputs because of his blindness, and because of the injuries and operations on his legs (joint replacements result in a loss of the body sensation from the joint). He also had a peripheral neuropathy.

- His ability to integrate this information in the brain was affected by his strokes and by cerebral small vessel disease (seen on his brain scan).

- He had weakness of both legs, because of his previous injuries, his cerebrovascular disease, and deconditioning.

- He had long-standing disability because of his previous accident.

He had managed very well with all this, until a new injury—a torn Achilles tendon—was simply more than his system could cope with, and he started to fall. He lost confidence and became reluctant to walk, losing more strength as a result.

He had a prolonged period of rehabilitation, but made little progress, and became more immobile. Eventually he had to be looked after in a care home.

6

Difficulty in walking and poor gait

> ## → Key points

> ◆ Walking becomes slower and less secure with age.

> ◆ Previous injuries, arthritis of joints, and muscular weakness cause difficulty walking in later life.

> ◆ Neurological disease—Parkinson's disease, stroke, small vessel disease, and many others—causes abnormal gaits that lead to falls.

Most falls occur on initially standing up, while walking, or on turning round. Those that occur immediately on getting out of a chair or bed are most commonly due to postural giddiness and unsteadiness (often due to drops in blood pressure (see Chapter 9)). Falls which occur while walking can have many causes.

Many falls are the result of stumbles that occur while walking. A younger person would be able to prevent a fall because of quicker reflexes and stronger legs, but an older person falls. With increasing age the number of stumbles increases. The chance that any given stumble will become a fall is also greater. There are many reasons for this.

There are changes in walking that come on with age. With increasing age people tend to stop and stand still when they want to talk. Those who have to do so are at increased risk of falling, because it is something that people start to do when their walking is less secure. Diverting attention from walking to talking makes them feel unsafe on their feet. The brain no longer has the reserves to cope with both tasks.

As people grow older they tend to have a natural pace that is slower. They may still be able to walk quickly, but left to decide for themselves they walk sedately. They tend to take shorter steps, and tend to spend more time with both feet on the ground, lifting the back foot less promptly as the weight goes onto the front foot. These are the natural adjustments that might be expected in someone who wanted to make their walking safer and more secure. In general, fallers tend to walk more slowly than non-fallers.

Many falls are related to trips and stumbles. Often poor vision, or distortion from bifocal or varifocal spectacles, contributes to these. Fallers have greater difficulty (compared with non-fallers) in navigating obstacles. They do so more slowly and with less precision. If there is an obstacle, they are more likely to touch it accidentally with their foot. In order to make the movements to avoid it, they have to break their step, and are unable to incorporate these obstacles into their normal walking pattern.

With advancing age, long-standing minor problems, which have never before caused a problem with walking, start to cause difficulties. The 'spare capacity' in the balance system has gone, and what was a minor nuisance now causes disability. The old footballing injury, the broken leg in your teens that never healed properly, the abnormal hip not properly treated when you were an infant, or just the lifelong tendency to not pick your feet up properly—any of these can start to cause walking difficulties leading to falls in later life.

Arthritis is a common cause of muscular weakness, and causes joints to give way. It affects walking by causing an abnormal gait. It causes changes in standing and gait to protect the painful joint. This change in posture may affect balance and posture, and impair the way the body can change its position in response to being put off balance

In addition, specific diseases will affect walking. Probably the most common is arthritis of the hips, knees, and ankles. The normal strategies for making fine movements to adjust balance at the ankles and hips will be impaired. It will also cause weakness in the muscles surrounding the joint, and the pain may cause a tendency for the joint to give way. Such weakness will also make falls more likely in those who are losing weight and becoming frail with increasing age.

📄 Case history

George was a 92-year-old man who had started to fall in the last 4 months. He was now falling several times every day. He had no warning, but just toppled over as he walked.

He had no cardiac disease, and was taking no medications. He had a moderate dementia. He lived with his wife.

No specific neurological or cardiovascular cause was found for his falls. When he walked, he placed his feet carelessly and inappropriately, so that when he transferred his weight onto the front foot, he was in an unstable position and fell. This was attributed to his dementia.

Reluctantly he agreed to use a wheeled frame, and by leaning on this as he walked he could do so more safely. Unfortunately, his wife reported that he would not use it in the house and his falls continued. He had no insight into his problem, no memory of having a problem with his walking, and no carry over following repeated sessions with the physiotherapist.

Sadly, not all falls can be prevented. His wife benefited from education about the cause of his falls and how he should be managed.

Stroke will cause difficulty walking in a number of ways. Patients who have had a paralysed leg may find that the leg remains weak and unable to bear their weight fully. Perhaps the leg might not be able to straighten fully when the weight is on it, or might have a tendency to give way. The different muscle groups in the leg may have difficulty coordinating their actions. In addition, on swinging the bad leg through during walking, it may not clear the ground as well as the good leg, resulting in a tendency to catch on the ground or on obstacles.

In its later stages, Parkinson's disease causes abnormal walking, with slow short shuffling steps. Often step length is uneven, and the feet are not picked up high enough off the ground. The posture is abnormal, with a tendency to lean forward. This causes the centre of gravity to be further forward over the front part of the feet, so that walking consists of rapid small steps to catch up with it. Patients with Parkinson's disease look as though they are hurrying after something, and the diagnosis is often first suspected because of their abnormal gait.

Falls in Parkinson's disease and related conditions occur for a number of reasons. The condition itself causes postural instability, and also orthostatic hypotension in some cases. Because of the combination of the rigidity of the body, the centre of gravity being in the wrong place, and the slow and impaired response to anything that challenges balance, falls are common.

Another cause of falling specific to Parkinson's disease is freezing of movement. As the patient tries to make a movement, they adjust their weight to anticipate it. They freeze, and the movement does not happen. They have already shifted their weight, and are now in an unstable position. They cannot return to their previous position quickly enough, lose balance, and topple over.

Small vessel disease of the brain may lead to a clinical picture that is often confused with Parkinson's disease. Typically, there are short steps, and a slow stiff gait. It is frequently difficult to distinguish between these two conditions, and often only a trial of treatment for Parkinson's disease will clarify the situation.

Patients with conditions affecting the cerebellum often complain that they walk as though they are drunk. Some are reluctant to leave the house because of what people will think of them. The limbs are not coordinated, and they may stagger from one side to the other like a drunken sailor. They are obviously off balance, and moments will occur when they cannot correct their position quickly enough, resulting in falls.

Foot drop

When the muscles at the front of the lower leg become weak or paralysed, the foot drops down as the leg is picked up, so that the toes drop forward towards the ground. There are several causes for this, including strokes and trapped nerves in the spine. One common cause is damage to a nerve (the common peroneal nerve) leading to the foot. This nerve curls round the bone at the outside of the leg just below the knee, where it is very vulnerable to injury.

If there is a foot drop, the foot tends to drag, and is more likely to catch on the ground during walking. It is treated with splints that are worn inside the shoes to help hold the foot up.

7

What causes giddiness?

 Key points

Giddiness:

- is a very complex and poorly understood symptom

- when it occurs on standing, can be caused by a drop in the blood supply to the brain

- occurs when the brain has insufficient information to tell it where it is in space

- is strongly associated with anxiety and depression

- is a common side effect of medications

- needs to be distinguished from vertigo.

Where no treatable cause is found, coping strategies help people to manage their problem.

Giddiness and unsteadiness are the symptoms most commonly associated with falls. It is very difficult for patients to describe these symptoms, and in particular it is often difficult to distinguish from the patient's story whether they have giddiness or vertigo—words that are often used interchangeably, even by doctors.

What is meant by giddiness? It is something we have all experienced during colds or influenza, or during sinus infections. We have all experienced giddiness caused by standing up too quickly.

A variety of words are used to describe giddiness. People say that they are giddy, dizzy, muzzy headed, or feel fuzzy or fuggy. In some cases there is unsteadiness without giddiness, and this is particularly difficult for some people to put into words. The symptoms of dizziness are slightly different for each patient. It can be momentary, as when you stand up or turn round suddenly. It can be prolonged and persistent, and not go away when you sit down. It is commonly associated with a sensation of being unsteady, and a desire to sit down.

What is giddiness?

Giddiness is a normal phenomenon. It occurs when, for some reason, the brain is not content with the amount of information it is receiving about its position. It could be described as the brain's distress signal when it is unable to assess where it is in space.

There are several potential causes for this. One is that the brain is not receiving sufficient information from the nerves of body sensation to form a judgement about its position in space. Another is that the brain might also be unable to interpret information because of the effects of medications, or because it has been damaged by small vessel disease, strokes, head injuries, or one of many other disease processes affecting the brain. Thirdly, the information that is being received may not be interpreted properly because the brain is not functioning normally because of a sudden reduction in its blood supply due to changes in blood pressure on standing. Frequently, more than one of these three things occurs at the same time.

The situations in which giddiness occurs most often are on standing up from a chair and on turning round. Both of these situations lead to a sudden but short-lived drop in the amount of sensory information reaching the brain. Movement leads to a change in the sensory input coming from nerves in muscles, joints, and tendons. At the same time, the balance organ in the inner ear takes a second or two to accustom itself to its new position. As the head is turned, there is a brief moment before the eyes fix upon what is in front of them during which time the brain is receiving reduced information about position from the eyes. Faced with the combined effect of these sudden changes and the reduction in sensory information, the brain sends out its distress signal—giddiness.

On standing up the change is even greater. Although visual information might change little and there is no rotational change in the inner ear, the change in information from the limbs, which is the most important in determining position in space, is greater. When sitting, a large part of the body's surface is in contact with a solid surface, and there is plenty of sensory information for the brain to work on. The feet, the backs of the thighs, the bottom, the back, and possibly the arms are supported. Suddenly, on standing up, all this information is lost except that from the feet. The result is giddiness.

Postural giddiness

The most common type of giddiness is that which occurs on standing up, particularly first thing in the morning or on getting out of bed. This is called postural giddiness. It is most often due to orthostatic hypotension (a drop in blood pressure that occurs on standing).

Postural giddiness is strongly related to orthostatic hypotension in the minds of many doctors and nurses, but the relationship is not as strong as many imagine. About a third of people with postural giddiness do not have significant orthostatic hypotension. People with giddiness from any other cause are also likely to have giddiness made worse by standing up, for reasons explained below.

Persistent giddiness

Some people have dizziness that persists even when they sit down or lie flat. Such giddiness is a great nuisance in that it tends to be there much of the time, and nothing really makes it better. For some people it is a life sentence. Typically it will be relieved by sleep, and will come on an hour or two after getting up in the morning. Occasionally people are giddy just on moving their eyes. This means that the problem must lie in the brain or the inner ear. Sometimes it is brought on by lying down flat. Some people are unable to lie flat in bed because doing so makes them giddy.

Persistent giddiness of this type is usually caused by the brain being affected by diffuse disease of the blood vessels (termed small vessel disease), which is common in people with high blood pressure, diabetes, or atrial fibrillation (an irregular chaotic heart rhythm). It can also be due to the side effects of certain drugs. Occasionally this sort of giddiness is seen in people who started with vertigo, but whose brain has adjusted to it, and now produces giddiness instead of a sensation of movement.

📄 Case history

Phyllis was an 84-year-old woman who had fallen four times in the previous 3 months, and who had persistent giddiness. The giddiness was present all the time, but much worse on getting out of a chair. She slept on four pillows at night, and was unable to lie flat because it made her feel giddy.

She had a long history of heart disease, with an irregular pulse (atrial fibrillation). She was a diet-controlled diabetic, and had high blood pressure that was poorly controlled.

She took three different tablets for her blood pressure. She had mild orthostatic hypotension, but her giddiness was not improved by altering her tablets.

A brain scan showed that she had extensive small vessel disease, and this was probably the cause of her symptoms. Treatment involved medication to control her blood pressure and to diminish the chances of a stroke with aspirin and a statin. She attended one of our balance and safety courses to teach her coping strategies, and to help her to come to terms with her disability. Her medication was adjusted so that she did not have orthostatic hypotension, and she had no more falls.

The situation in real life is more complex. The changes above may take place in someone who may also, at the same moment, be experiencing a sudden drop in the blood supply to the brain due to orthostatic hypotension, may have poor vision, and may have chronic changes in the brain, which mean that the ability to make sense of the information available is impaired.

What can be done about giddiness?

- **Take things slowly** By persuading the patient to do things more slowly, the rate of change of sensory inputs is changed to a pace that the brain may cope with more easily.

- **Additional support and equipment** The uncertainty that comes with movement can be improved by using the arms for support—by making use of grab rails and walking frames. These also improve things by giving additional sensory information. The main function of a walking stick is to give additional sensory information from the hand about position in space, rather than to be a physical support.

- **Blood pressure** That part of giddiness that is due to orthostatic hypotension may improve if the drop in blood pressure can be diminished. This could be by changing some medications, or by other specific treatments.

Where there is an element of giddiness due to chronic changes in the brain or vestibular system, little can be done to improve the situation. Treatment is aimed at preventing progression of the underlying disease, usually the control of high blood pressure.

◆ **Treat anxiety** Giddiness also has a significant psychological element. Anxiety related to confidence and security in performing movements causes giddiness or makes it worse. This can be improved with exercise classes and balance groups, discussed elsewhere.

Occasionally patients who say they have had long-standing giddiness turn out to have had vertigo when their problem started. The vertigo may have stopped years ago, leaving just giddiness. This is important, because the diagnosis is one of a condition that causes vertigo, which differs from the list of conditions that cause only giddiness.

8

What is vertigo?

⟹ Key points

◆ The most common cause of vertigo among fallers is benign positional vertigo (BPV). This is the only cause of vertigo that can be cured easily.

◆ Vestibular neuronitis and Ménière's disease are common causes in younger people.

◆ Other causes of vertigo are less common, and include strokes affecting the brainstem and cerebellum, migraine, tumours of the vestibular nerve, and other causes of damage to the vestibular system.

The main feature distinguishing vertigo from giddiness is a feeling of sudden movement, particularly rotation. The sensation is described as being like that caused by spinning round and round and then stopping suddenly, or stepping off a roundabout that has been going round quickly. For most people this is an experience they remember from childhood, but many people find this sensation difficult to put into words.

It can be a very distressing symptom, which can come on suddenly and violently, causing the patient to fall, or to feel very unwell with severe nausea or vomiting. Attacks can be brought on by movements of the head, or even by moving the eyes. Episodes occur unpredictably, and are disabling. Between attacks, the patient may be completely well or may have persistent unsteadiness or giddiness on movement.

What causes vertigo?

Vertigo is usually caused by abnormal information sent from the inner ear on one side, which gives chaotic information to the brain about where the head is in space. Because the information is unbalanced—normal on one side and abnormal on the other—the brain interprets it as though the head is spinning round (even though it is not). Under such circumstances, it is very difficult to maintain balance if the attack starts while standing.

Normally, the brain adjusts to the abnormal signals coming from the inner ear after a few weeks or months and stops responding by causing vertigo, but may cause giddiness instead. In such cases the diagnosis may be difficult unless specific questions are asked about episodes of vertigo, which may well have been forgotten by the patient.

In some cases, vertigo can arise as a result of diseases of the nerve to the ear, or the connections to that nerve within the brain. Conditions such as stroke, particularly in the cerebellum and the brainstem, can cause persistent symptoms of unsteadiness or vertigo.

♦ **Vestibular neuronitis** The most common cause of vertigo in the general population is a viral infection that affects the inner ear, called vestibular neuronitis. This unpleasant condition may go on for weeks, and may cause lasting damage to the nerve which can cause symptoms in later life. In the short term, the symptoms recover spontaneously, but may be suppressed by medication.

♦ **Ménière's disease** is a condition of middle age which causes deafness and tinnitus (a persistent whining noise in the ears), together with episodes of vertigo. It is unusual for this condition to start at the age at which people start to experience unexplained falls, and it tends to be diagnosed in error fairly frequently. There is a drug treatment for Ménière's disease, which does not work for other forms of vertigo, and many GPs give patients a trial of this to see if it has any effect. There is some debate about its efficacy in Ménière's disease.

♦ **Benign positional vertigo** In the age group at which people start to have recurrent falls the usual cause of vertigo is 'benign positional vertigo'. In later life this is a more common cause of vertigo than either Ménière's disease or vestibular neuronitis, accounting for about half the total. Characteristically, this is vertigo brought on by movements of the head. It tends to be one particular movement in any particular patient, but the most common by far is vertigo caused by turning over in bed. Benign positional vertigo is caused by small pieces of chalk in the inner ear, called otoliths, becoming displaced and travelling down the semicircular canals, where they give rise to abnormal signals which cause vertigo. The diagnosis is made on the history and on the response to treatment. There is a quick and simple treatment, called Epley's manoeuvre, which involves putting the patient into certain positions for 30 seconds at a time. Epley's manoeuvre positions each semicircular canal in turn into a position that encourages the otoliths to fall back into their correct place. It is harmless, and can be repeated as often as necessary if the symptoms recur. It is successful in relieving symptoms in 70–80 per cent of cases (Figure 8.1). The patient can be taught to do the manoeuvre at home. Symptoms commonly recur. About a third of patients will have a recurrence within a year, and about half will have further symptoms in the next 5 years.

Often it is unclear what the cause of the vertigo might be until the patient has had an Epley's manoeuvre on clinical suspicion that the diagnosis is benign positional vertigo. If the symptoms improve, the diagnosis was correct. Some people recommend that patients should sleep semi-upright for 2 days after an Epley's manoeuvre. They should avoid lying on the affected side, and avoid the movements that bring on symptoms. It is not clear whether this really makes any difference.

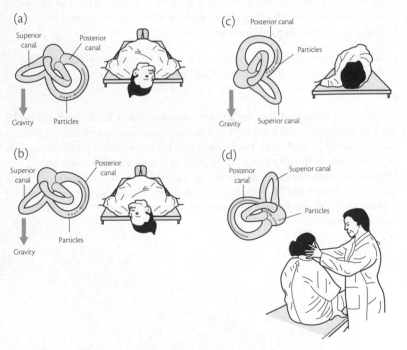

Figure 8.1 Epley's manoeuvre.

Many patients have a history of vertigo, and have a degree of persistent damage to their vestibular system, usually caused by previous viral labyrinthitis. Eventually the brain readjusts to the signals from the damaged ear, but it may not do so fully. The inner ear may become abnormally sensitive to movement, and not give accurate information about position. If the damage is on one side, it may alter the brain's perception of where vertical is, and this may result in inappropriate rebalancing movements that put the patient off balance.

📄 Case history

Jane was an 82-year-old woman who had a history of giddiness related to head movement and posture for about 2 years. On repeated questioning, she eventually remembered that this had started with her having episodes of vertigo when lying in bed. Whenever she turned over in bed to the left side she developed vertigo. The symptoms had now evolved into giddiness on head movement, but she still had occasional vertigo.

She had an Epley's manoeuvre, and during this developed intense vertigo and nystagmus, confirming the diagnosis of benign positional vertigo. This cured her of her giddiness and vertigo.

Subsequently some milder symptoms returned about 4 months later, but these were also cured with a repeat of Epley's manoeuvre.

Occasionally patients have vertigo due to causes other than inner ear problems. It may be the first symptom of a benign tumour affecting the nerve from the ear (acoustic neuroma), particularly if it is accompanied by deafness. It is normal practice to carry out a brain scan in patients with vertigo where the cause is not immediately clear. Vertigo can also arise from damage to the back part of the brain—the brainstem and cerebellum. This is commonly caused by a small stroke. In such cases the symptoms usually improve over time, but do not always resolve completely.

9

How can the heart and circulation contribute to falls?

> ### ⮕ Key points
>
> Giddiness, falls, and loss of consciousness can be caused by:
>
> - Conditions that cause low blood pressure:
>
>   - orthostatic hypotension
>
>   - simple faints (vasovagal syndrome)
>
>   - vasodepressor carotid sinus hypersensitivity
>
>   - treatments that reduce blood pressure.
>
> - Conditions that affect the pulse:
>
>   - a pulse that is rapid—supraventricular tachycardia, rapid atrial fibrillation
>
>   - a pulse that is ineffective—ventricular tachycardia
>
>   - a pulse that is too slow—complete heart block
>
>   - a pulse that has prolonged pauses—sick sinus syndrome, cardio-inhibitory carotid sinus hypersensitivity.
>
> Where these conditions are the cause of falls, a diagnosis is important because they are all treatable conditions, and will recur until they are treated successfully.

Among those who have had a fall during which they might have lost consciousness, and those who have had recurrent unexplained falls, it is probable that there is some underlying medical cause. While there are many causes of brief loss of consciousness, the two most common are derangements of the pulse or blood pressure. Until this is diagnosed and treated, the falls or loss of consciousness are likely to recur.

> An abnormality of the pulse or blood pressure leading to a drop in blood supply to the brain is the most common medical reason contributing to falls. It is found in about 40 per cent of patients seen in the clinic.

A sudden reduction in the blood supply to the brain may last for only a few seconds, or may go on for several minutes. It is sufficient to cause brief unconsciousness, or unsteadiness and an inability to retain balance.

Passing out as a result of reduced blood supply to the brain is termed syncope (pronounced sin-kerpy, which translates roughly from the Greek as 'a pause' in consciousness). Feeling giddy or unsteady because of a fall in blood supply to the brain is termed pre-syncope.

These conditions are often caused, or made worse, by a variety of commonly used medicines (see Chapter 10). These medicines are normally prescribed for good reasons, and are most commonly very appropriate medicines for the patient to have and well tolerated by most people. However, as with all medications, a percentage of people do develop side effects.

Blood pressure

A drop in blood pressure is a common cause of falls. There are several common mechanisms leading to a drop in blood pressure that can cause giddiness, falls, or loss of consciousness:

- medications that reduce the blood pressure

- orthostatic hypotension

- simple faints (vasovagal syndrome)

- vasodepressor carotid sinus hypersensitivity

- coughing

- straining on the toilet.

Medications

Many people take medication that affects the pulse or blood pressure for years, and have no side effects. In a small proportion of people, ability to tolerate these tablets diminishes over time. If they continue with the tablets, the blood pressure may be reduced far too much, leading to giddiness, falls, and faints. Simply cutting back the dose or stopping the medication altogether may be enough to prevent further symptoms.

Orthostatic hypotension (also called postural hypotension)

> ➲ Key points
>
> - Affects about 15 per cent of people aged over 75 years.
>
> - Is usually asymptomatic.
>
> - Can cause giddiness or unsteadiness on standing or walking.
>
> - Is defined as a drop of 20 mmHg in systolic pressure or 10 mmHg in diastolic pressure from lying to standing.
>
> - Is the most common cardiovascular cause of falls and loss of consciousness.
>
> - Can be caused by medications.
>
> - Vitamin B_{12} deficiency is an important cause because it is easily cured.
>
> - In the absence of vitamin B_{12} deficiency or a causative medication it is difficult to treat, but the symptoms can be managed.

This is the most common medical cause of giddiness, falls, and loss of consciousness in people aged over 75 years. Orthostatic hypotension means a significant drop in blood pressure on standing.

It is common for the blood pressure to drop on standing in certain situations, and this happens to everyone from time to time. This does not cause any symptoms in most people,, and they are completely unaware of it. In some people it causes giddiness on standing, and in a small minority it causes them to fall or to pass out.

Normally, blood pressure changes very little when one stands up. It can go up or down slightly. In many older people the systems controlling blood pressure do not work properly, and the blood pressure drops by a significant amount on standing, but few of them are troubled by it.

What is 'a significant amount'? There is an enormous difference between one person and another in the drops in blood pressure that are required to produce symptoms, and most people who meet the criteria for having orthostatic hypotension do not have any symptoms. In one study, one in seven people aged over 75 years was found to have a significant drop in blood pressure on standing, although only one in 50 admitted to any giddiness, and a much smaller number had passed out.

When orthostatic hypotension does cause symptoms, these usually consist of giddiness or unsteadiness on standing up. Less commonly, the giddiness occurs some time after first getting up. Typically, falls happen immediately on getting out of a chair, or on getting out of bed in the middle of the night (with or without the giddiness). Uncommonly orthostatic hypotension is so severe that sitting up causes loss of consciousness.

Most people who fall because of orthostatic hypotension have episodes of giddiness, usually associated with their fall, but also at other times. In some people falls due to orthostatic hypotension can occur without giddiness.

When orthostatic hypotension does cause giddiness, it goes away on sitting down again and there is no giddiness when lying flat in bed. If the giddiness persists on lying flat, it has a different cause.

What causes orthostatic hypotension?

When one stands up blood drains downwards within the body. It pools in large veins in the legs and lower abdomen. In order to get this blood back to the heart to be pumped round the circulation normally, these blood vessels must constrict to squeeze the blood upwards again. If the blood stays pooled in the legs and abdomen, the body has effectively lost some of its circulating volume, less blood is pumped by the heart, and the blood pressure drops.

The blood vessels are surrounded by thin sheets of muscle fibre which constrict when they are stimulated by nerves. When these muscle sheets are made to contract, they squeeze the blood vessels, causing blood to be forced back towards the heart. Anything that affects the working of the nerves is likely to result in difficulty in returning blood to the heart, and therefore in maintaining the blood pressure in an upright position.

In this condition, the circulation is very similar to a balloon half full of water. When it is lying flat the whole balloon is filled with water. On picking up one end, water drains from the upper part, and can only be forced back there by squeezing the lower part of the balloon.

This type of drop in blood pressure is common in people who are ill. Any factor that reduces the amount of blood in the circulation can cause orthostatic hypotension. Anything that results in a fever, or which causes the patient to become dehydrated, either through not wanting to drink or by fluid loss from bleeding, vomiting, or diarrhoea, can cause it.

A large variety of medicines can cause orthostatic hypotension as a side effect. These medicines are well tolerated by most people, but they may result in a drop in blood pressure in those who are susceptible, particularly when they are unwell.

Some people have severe and symptomatic orthostatic hypotension all the time. In some the cause is clear. These include patients with Parkinson's disease or conditions resembling it, in which those parts of the brain that control blood pressure are affected by the disease. Persistent orthostatic hypotension can also be caused by diabetes, which damages the nerves to blood vessels. Vitamin B_{12} deficiency, too much alcohol, peripheral neuropathy, and any other condition that leads to damaged nerves will also cause it.

Some women with a tendency to urinary incontinence tend not to drink a great deal, so as not to make their incontinence worse. This can lead to long-term dehydration, which appears to be a common cause of orthostatic hypotension.

Orthostatic hypotension is commonly found in people who have high blood pressure (hypertension). It has been found that about a third of people with poorly controlled high blood pressure, or people who have untreated high blood pressure, have orthostatic hypotension. Most of these people will have no symptoms. The reason for this link between high blood pressure and a tendency for the blood pressure to drop on standing is not understood. It is believed that there is some abnormality in the body's blood pressure control systems.

In some people an underlying cause for this condition is never found, and it appears to be something they are affected by for no clear reason. It is assumed that there has been an age-related deterioration in the nerves to the blood vessels, but there has been little research to prove this.

Symptoms in orthostatic hypotension

The severity of symptoms in orthostatic hypotension is very variable. While most people may be unaware they have this condition, others are so severely affected that they are unable to sit up without losing consciousness.

Characteristically, patients with orthostatic hypotension will have periods of giddiness or unsteadiness on first getting out of a chair. It is possible that they will not experience giddiness, but will simply collapse back into the chair or fall onto the floor. Others have no symptoms, but simply collapse while walking around the house or out in the street. These episodes of collapse may or may not be associated with loss of consciousness. If they are, the patient usually regains consciousness very quickly after they have hit the floor.

Other symptoms include fatigue, weakness, and changes in vision, which typically 'tunnels' or blacks out when the blood pressure has dropped a long way. Patients may feel vague or muddled. There may be a dull aching pain across the back of the shoulders, in what is termed a 'coat hanger' distribution. There may be a similar pain in the lower back or buttocks.

Case history

William was a 76-year-old man who had been on treatment for high blood pressure for 20 years. He was referred because he had three unexplained falls, when his legs 'just gave way'. He said that he had never had any giddiness or lost consciousness.

He was taking lisinopril 30 mg a day. His blood pressure was 130/70 mmHg lying and 90/60 mmHg standing, without symptoms of giddiness. His lisinopril was stopped and he had no further falls. He was treated with losartan 50 mg a day, and on review his blood pressure was 128/76 mmHg both lying and standing.

Cases like this are common. About 60 per cent of older people taking lisinopril develop orthostatic hypotension. Several different types of medicine can cause this response, particularly some of those used for depression or to treat high blood pressure.

Diagnosing orthostatic hypotension

Orthostatic hypotension is diagnosed by measuring the lying and standing blood pressure. This means that the blood pressure is measured in the upper arm with the patient lying flat, and then measured again standing up.

This standing measurement is repeated several times over the first few minutes. Orthostatic hypotension is said to occur when the blood pressure falls by a certain amount. This fall can vary greatly in its timing. In most cases the fall occurs over the first few seconds, and then after a minute or two the blood pressure rises slightly to a new but lower level. In other cases the blood pressure sags over a few minutes.

An international committee has defined orthostatic hypotension as being a drop of 20 mmHg in the systolic blood pressure (upper number) or a drop of 10 mmHg in the diastolic pressure (lower number). In practical terms, in older patients, it is a drop in the systolic pressure that is found most commonly, and that is most significant. The lower reading (diastolic) changes little, if at all.

Many doctors and nurses use automatic blood pressure machines rather than the older means of listening with a stethoscope over the artery. Such machines take some time to generate readings, limiting the number of readings they can give, and are unlikely to give a reasonable estimate of the drop in blood pressure on standing.

An alternative method of measuring orthostatic hypotension is by putting the patient on a tilt table, which is an examination couch on a hinge, and tilting the patient up until they are nearly standing. This gives the same blood pressure drop as getting up from a bed, but because it is done to the patient without them having to move themselves, it is easier to make accurate measurements. Some people are unsteady when they first stand up and need to grab hold of things, which limits our ability to measure their blood pressure in the crucial first minute or two.

Treatment of orthostatic hypotension

The treatment of orthostatic hypotension is difficult. It consists of treating underlying factors such as anaemia, dehydration, vitamin B_{12} deficiency, or infection.

In many cases medication causes the orthostatic hypotension or makes it worse. The problem is that these medications are often necessary to treat other medical problems. Substituting them with alternatives that have a different side-effect profile may diminish the orthostatic hypotension, but there is little information available on which medications should be avoided and which should be used.

If orthostatic hypotension occurs during an illness, it may improve as the illness is treated and the patient's general condition improves. If it is due to dehydration, simply giving enough fluids, either by mouth, or if necessary through a drip, may be enough to restore the blood pressure more nearly to normal.

In a small number of cases orthostatic hypotension is treated with medicines to increase the blood pressure. For many people nothing resolves the problem entirely, and they have to learn to manage the problem and live with it.

Fludrocortisone

In cases where there does not seem to be a significant treatable underlying disorder, there are treatments that may improve the orthostatic hypotension. The medication that is used most frequently is called fludrocortisone. This acts on the kidney to cause a degree of salt and fluid retention, and leads to a slight increase in the amount of water in the circulation. This may correct the blood pressure abnormality, but does so in only a small percentage of cases. Some patients feel that their giddiness is a little better on this medication, but in very many cases it has no significant effect.

Its main side effects are indigestion and ankle swelling. It can also cause a drop in the level of potassium in the blood, which needs to be monitored. Very rarely, in those with heart failure, it can cause fluid to collect on the lungs and cause shortness of breath, in which case it should be stopped immediately.

Although fludrocortisone is a steroid, it is not the sort of steroid that causes loss of calcium from the bones or thinning of the skin. Pharmacists give instructions that it is not to be discontinued suddenly, which do not apply when it is being used to treat orthostatic hypotension. (Its main use is in Addison's disease, a failure of the adrenal gland to produce steroids, when it would be dangerous to stop it suddenly.)

The action of fludrocortisone is to reduce the amount of sodium lost in the urine. When sodium is retained, water will be retained with it, leading to an increase in the blood volume. The same effect can be achieved by taking salt tablets.

Midodrine

The second line of treatment is a tablet called midodrine. This is more effective, but there is some concern over potential side effects. This medicine is widely available in most countries except the UK, where the expense of producing research to prove its safety to satisfy the regulatory authorities is not justified by the small amount prescribed. It is available by special arrangement, and needs to be imported. The risks of its use are significant, but we do not know how large they are, and it is only prescribed by specialists.

Midodrine increases the blood pressure by activating the muscles around large veins causing them to squeeze the veins, thereby increasing the return of blood to the heart. It increases the blood pressure and reduces the extent of orthostatic hypotension. It is very effective in certain groups of patients—those with alcohol-related autonomic neuropathy do best—but less effective in others, such as those with Parkinson's or similar diseases (e.g. multi-system atrophy).

📄 Case history

John was an 82-year-old retired publican. He had drunk alcohol to excess throughout his adult life, and admitted to drinking half a bottle of vodka a day. He had collapsed in the kitchen, possibly with loss of consciousness. He had been conscious in the ambulance, but muddled (which was new for him). His confusion settled over a few days with antibiotic treatment of a urinary infection.

On the day after admission, the nurses sat him up in bed and he fainted. His blood pressure was 130/75 mmHg lying, but on sitting fell to 80/50 mmHg. On one occasion he was stood up between two people, and no blood pressure could be detected. He had to be laid flat again promptly.

His inability to sit up was due to severe orthostatic hypotension, probably as a consequence of his alcoholism. He was treated with midodrine, which was gradually increased to maximum doses. His condition improved dramatically. Within a few days his blood pressure was 140/80 mmHg lying and 90/60 mmHg standing, and once he was on maximum doses of midodrine, it was 150/90 mmHg both lying and standing. He was now independently mobile and had no postural giddiness.

He was followed up regularly for the next 3 years, during which time he gradually deteriorated in the way one might expect with age. Eventually he was admitted to hospital with a major stroke, leaving him severely paralysed down the right side and barely conscious. Over the next few days his condition deteriorated and he died.

Midodrine had clearly given him 3 years of useful good quality life, when other treatments would not have worked. The question remains as to what role it may have played in causing his stroke. We know that reducing the blood pressure reduces the risk of stroke. Presumably the opposite is true—that increasing the blood pressure increases the risk of stroke. And yet there are situations when this is the only course of action open to us.

There is a lack of data about the safety of this medication. I use midodrine very sparingly, and only when everything else has been considered or tried.

Hypertension with orthostatic hypotension

High blood pressure is very common with advancing age. In about a third of people with untreated hypertension it goes hand in hand with orthostatic hypotension. The reason for this is not clear, but there does seem to be some fundamental derangement of blood pressure control.

In a small minority of patients restoring the high blood pressure to normal leads to resolution of the orthostatic hypotension. In the majority of patients, when these two conditions occur together, neither of them will generate any symptoms. However, there are patients who develop symptoms of orthostatic hypotension as soon as their hypertension is treated.

The aim of treatment is to have a stable and steady blood pressure with resolution of the patient's symptoms of postural giddiness. This can often be achieved by careful attempts to select the right medications for that patient. Ultimately, falls are a greater and more immediate risk than high blood pressure, and if the falls are due to problems with the blood pressure, treatment should be kept to a minimum.

📄 Case history

Elizabeth was a 72-year-old woman who was referred after she suddenly passed out and fell, breaking her right wrist. For the last 8 years she had noticed giddiness and unsteadiness on getting up suddenly. She had had one other episode of collapse about 3 months earlier, when she had got up in the night to go to the toilet.

Her blood pressure was 180/80 mmHg lying and 120/76 mmHg standing, with unsteadiness on standing. This was confirmed on three separate occasions.

She had never before been noted to have high blood pressure. She was treated with losartan, gradually increased to 50 mg/day, and with fludrocortisone 0.1 mg/day, and her symptoms improved. Her blood pressure was 140/80 mmHg lying and 130/80 mmHg standing, with no symptoms on standing.

She remained well with a stable blood pressure and no falls or giddiness for the following year. She developed some ankle swelling, which is a common side effect of fludrocortisone (and which shows that it is having the desired effect of causing fluid retention).

The treatment of orthostatic hypotension in people with high blood pressure is problematic. Little research has been done in this field. It is desirable to reduce the high blood pressure, but treating it often makes the symptoms of orthostatic hypotension worse. The treatment is poorly tolerated and is often abandoned.

The addition of treatment for orthostatic hypotension often leads to a reduction in the drop in blood pressure on standing, and in many cases a satisfactory balance between blood pressure control and orthostatic symptoms can be achieved.

Living with orthostatic hypotension

For many people there is no effective remedy, and they have to go through their lives with symptoms of orthostatic hypotension. Everyone who has symptoms can benefit from planning their activities in such a way as to keep these symptoms to a minimum.

When symptoms do occur, most people want to sit down. Once sitting down, crossing the legs will increase the blood pressure for a few moments, and may be helpful.

If outside, sitting on a bench or a wall for a few minutes might allow symptoms to settle. If there is nowhere to sit, then squatting down as though to tie shoelaces or looking in a bag may be sufficient to help until the symptoms improve. Great care needs to be taken when getting up from this position, possibly asking others for help, as getting up from squatting itself causes orthostatic hypotension.

Another trick to increase the blood pressure for a few moments is to stand leaning against something, with legs crossed. Then stand on tiptoes, and clench the buttock muscles.

For those who do pass out, family and friends should be warned that this might happen, and told what to do—lie the patient flat on the ground or on a sofa, and if possible raise the legs in the air. They should remove any hot drinks and sharp objects for safety. They should check the pulse and breathing, and call an ambulance if these are not right—the pulse will be weak, and may be difficult to find, but it will be present. It should start to become stronger as soon as the patient is lying flat.

Symptoms occur most frequently on standing up suddenly, on moving about, and during exercise. They are most common on first getting up in the morning (and tend to be better in the afternoon and evening). They also occur after meals or after drinking alcohol. They can be brought on by straining in the toilet, or by bending over to pick things up or to do the gardening. They will be made worse by dehydration, particularly on hot days. Hot baths and showers will provoke them (use a tepid bath or shower). Any illness will make symptoms worse.

Orthostatic hypotension is a common condition that frequently goes undiagnosed because it is not considered. Even when it is, insufficient care is taken in assessing the blood pressure, or it is measured with an automatic cuff, or measured sitting and standing, leading to an underestimation of its severity. It can be difficult or even impossible to treat, but many cases respond to withdrawal of offending medications and rehydration.

Simple faints (vasovagal syndrome)

➲ Key points

- ◆ Fainting is not an illness but a normal reflex that is exaggerated in some people.

- ◆ It may be a mechanism to deceive predators—'playing dead' is common in many animals.

- ◆ It is usually associated with symptoms before the fainting starts— sweating, nausea, lightheadedness, and feeling unwell.

- ◆ In some cases there is collapse with loss of consciousness without warning.

- ◆ It is diagnosed on the history in most cases, and by tilt testing when the diagnosis is unclear.

- ◆ It may be caused or made worse by medications.

- ◆ It is treated by withdrawal of causative medication or with fludrocortisone.

Fainting is part of common experience, particularly for young women, whose blood pressure is normally low. Most of us will have had times when we felt a little lightheaded. In some cases this can progress to a full-blown faint with collapse and possible loss of consciousness.

Commonly, fainting is accompanied by a feeling beforehand that tells us that something is not right. Giddiness, lightheadedness, or unsteadiness are most often accompanied by sweating, a feeling that the heart is thumping or racing (called palpitations), nausea, or even vomiting. Sometimes there are visual symptoms; typically patients say that things start to become distant and their vision starts to go dark or 'tunnel', and voices seem to recede into the distance.

While fainting in teenagers and young adults is common and expected, most of them grow out of it. Fainting starts to become a problem again in late middle age, and it is common in the elderly. It may run in the family. I often hear from younger patients that their mother used to faint at this age. Occasionally, patients who faint tell me that they have little or no salt in their food. Just increasing the amount of salt in the diet may be enough to stop them fainting.

Maintaining the blood pressure while in an upright posture depends on the action of the sympathetic nervous system, a system of small nerves acting on muscles around the blood vessels. There needs to be an increase in sympathetic activity on standing up, and the sympathetic system is put under a degree of stress. On more prolonged standing, this stress slowly increases as more and more blood pools in the large blood vessels of the legs and lower abdomen. With time, fluid starts to leak out of the circulation into the tissues, making the work of the sympathetic system harder still. Eventually, in susceptible people, a point is reached at which the sympathetic system has had enough and switches off.

The effect of this can be catastrophic, with a sudden drop in blood pressure, often associated with a marked slowing of the pulse. This is said to be the mechanism of a simple faint (also called vasovagal syndrome or neurocardiogenic syncope).

Vasovagal attacks are frequently caused by **medications**. Any medicine that opens up the blood vessels or diminishes the amount of water in the blood can provoke fainting. Typically, these are medications that are used for the treatment of high blood pressure, heart failure, or angina. These drugs are usually well tolerated, and do not cause these side effects in most patients. In most cases the choice of drug has been appropriate for the patient's condition.

The diagnosis of vasovagal syndrome is usually made on the basis of the history, and when nothing wrong is found with the patient in the clinic. There is a test, called the tilt test, which aims to provoke an attack while under observation and monitoring. The patient is put on a tilt table at 70–80°, i.e. almost

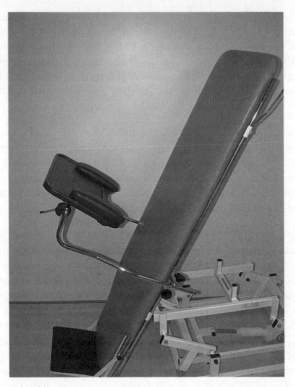

Figure 9.1 A tilt table.

standing, but leaning back slightly (Figure 9.1) and left in that position for up to 40 minutes. The normal response to this would be that there would be no change in blood pressure, or perhaps a slight drop over a 40-minute period, with no symptoms. In those in whom the test is positive, blood pressure may start to fluctuate a few minutes into the test and eventually begin to drop rapidly to a level at which the patient starts to have symptoms and may even lose consciousness.

📄 Case history

Freda was an 83-year-old woman with a long history of angina. One morning she developed tightness in the chest while out shopping. She put a glyceryl trinitrate (GTN) tablet under her tongue to treat this attack of angina.

After about a minute, she started to feel sweaty and nauseated. Her vision began to go dark, and she heard voices receding into the distance. She then collapsed to the floor unconscious, and an ambulance was called.

She had recovered by the time the ambulance arrived, and refused to come to hospital. She felt unwell for the rest of the day, but was back to her normal self by the next day.

GTN tablets or spray for angina are very common causes of fainting.

Tilt tests are very time consuming, and can make patients feel unwell. The results are not always clear. If someone has a normal test, they might still have vasovagal syndrome. About one in 20 normal people will have a positive tilt test in the absence of any previous symptoms. The results are difficult to interpret. Not surprisingly, few people have this test done.

Treatment of vasovagal syndrome

The first thing to remember about fainting is that it is not an illness, but a normal reflex. It does not necessarily require any treatment. When it is sufficiently frequent or severe to need treatment, this consists of withdrawing any offending medications and trying to substitute them with others that are less likely to cause this side effect. Where no medications are involved, treatment is with fludrocortisone, which tends to be more successful in older patients with this condition than in those with orthostatic hypotension. Unfortunately, no research has been done to determine exactly how effective it is, but many patients find that it makes them feel better and abolishes their attacks. Occasionally patients may find that adding more salt to their diet or taking salt tablets has a sufficient effect in terms of retaining fluid in the circulation to abolish the symptoms. Midodrine has been used in resistant cases, but again there are no data on how effective it is. Pacemakers have been used, but are usually of little benefit.

Living with vasovagal syndrome

Once the diagnosis of vasovagal syndrome has been established, a great deal of the anxiety about recurrent episodes of unconsciousness will be relieved. The problem is one of injuries sustained during falls. Usually the falls occur with some warning, and teaching the patient how to behave when they first feel the attack coming on can prevent the consequences of a fall. As soon as symptoms are felt, the patient should lie down if possible. If that is not practical, then they should sit down, and try the methods outlined above to increase blood pressure by crossing the legs and clenching the thigh muscles.

Carotid sinus hypersensitivity

➔ Key points

- Carotid sinus hypersensitivity (CSH) is a common cause of unexplained falls and syncope.

- It is due to excessive sensitivity of the nerves supplying the carotid sinus, part of the carotid artery in the neck.

- There are two forms, which can occur together as a mixed form.

- Cardio-inhibitory CSH leads to a pause in the pulse for a few seconds. It can be treated successfully with a pacemaker.

- Vasodepressor CSH causes a sudden drop in blood pressure lasting only a few seconds. It requires special equipment to establish the diagnosis. Like other conditions leading to a fall in blood pressure, it is made worse by many medications.

CSH is a common condition, which is often found in people who have lost consciousness or who have had unexplained falls. It affects about one in 20 older people but produces symptoms in only a few of them.

The carotid sinus is an area of widening of the carotid artery (Figure 9.2) just before it enters the bottom of the skull on its way to supply blood to the brain. It is densely supplied by nerves from the sympathetic system, and is involved in the control of blood pressure. In some people it becomes over-sensitive, and turning the head, looking up, or any activity that stretches the carotid artery can cause a profound drop in blood pressure or a prolonged pause in the pulse, sufficient to reduce blood flow to the brain. This can lead to unsteadiness, a fall, or even collapse with loss of consciousness. Frequently these symptoms occur without any obvious actions that might have stretched the neck.

There are two main forms of this condition. In **vasodepressor** syndrome there is a drop in blood pressure sufficient to cause a drop in blood flow to the brain. The other form, **cardio-inhibitory** syndrome, leads to a pause in the beating of the heart, which can be quite prolonged—in some cases up to 15 seconds. In the **mixed** form, both of these things occur together.

To test for carotid sinus hypersensitivity the patient is attached to an ECG machine and a finger blood pressure monitor. The carotid artery in the neck is rubbed quite firmly for about 10 seconds. If the result is negative, the test is

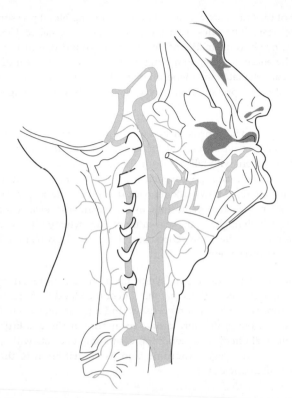

Figure 9.2 The carotid sinus.

repeated on the other side. This test is often done on a tilt table, and responses are more likely to be positive if the circulation is put under stress by tilting the patient up to between 70–80° for a few minutes.

To detect cardio-inhibitory carotid sinus syndrome an ECG is run during this procedure, and any pause in the pulse is visible on the tracing. A pause of more than 3 seconds is considered to be significant. Most people have some degree of slowing of the pulse on massaging the carotid sinus.

In patients who have vasodepressor carotid sinus syndrome the change in blood pressure is very rapid, and it returns to normal again very quickly. Typically, the whole of the drop in blood pressure is over in about 25 seconds. The usual methods of measuring blood pressure are not quick enough to measure such a change, and a special blood pressure machine must be used.

A number of machines are available that measure the blood pressure for each beat of the heart. The ones used most commonly are called Finapres and Portapres. They have a small cuff, which is put round one of the fingers. It measures the volume of blood entering the finger with each beat of the heart, and from that calculates the blood pressure. It is not particularly accurate as a measure of blood pressure, but is very good at showing changes in blood pressure.

Cardio-inhibitory syndrome is treated with a pacemaker. Recent studies have cast some doubt on the efficacy of this treatment, and the difficulty is determining which patient with falls is having them because of this condition, rather than from another cause. A pacemaker cures some people, but makes little difference for others. Many patients with this syndrome also have a variety of other problems (such as orthostatic hypotension, vasovagal syndrome, and arrhythmias) which might be the real cause of their syncope. These conditions are often found together, and represent a generalized problem affecting the autonomic nervous system.

The treatment of vasodepressor syndrome is much more difficult. Once again, cutting back medications that may affect the blood pressure helps some people. Treatments such as fludrocortisone and midodrine, used in other conditions in which blood pressure drops, are used, but there is little evidence of their beneficial effect. This condition commonly coexists with orthostatic hypotension and vasovagal syndrome, and its contribution to the patient's symptoms is often unclear.

📄 Case history

John was an 82-year-old man who was brought into hospital having collapsed in his kitchen. He had a history of two other episodes of passing out over the past year—one while sitting at dinner, and the other while weeding the garden.

When his right carotid artery was rubbed, his pulse stopped for 10 seconds and he passed out. The probable diagnosis was carotid sinus hypersensitivity. He had a pacemaker inserted and was discharged.

At follow-up he was started on ramipril because of impaired heart function. His GP was told to increase it gradually to 10 mg. He started to pass out again, but this ceased when the ramipril was withdrawn. The ramipril was substituted with valsartan. He remained well subsequently and had no more falls in the next 6 months.

Abnormal heart rhythms (arrhythmias)

Episodes of loss of consciousness can commonly be caused by a drop in blood pressure caused by abnormalities of the pulse rate. These fall into several categories:

◆ a pulse that is too rapid for the heart to fill sufficiently with blood between beats

◆ a pulse that is too slow to pump blood effectively

◆ an irregular pulse, with pauses between beats of 3 seconds or more resulting in a drop in blood flow to the brain.

Giddiness, unsteadiness, and loss of consciousness are usually the only symptoms of arrhythmias. There are two things in the patient's history which might provide a clue to the diagnosis. Firstly, the patient may already have an irregular pulse, or have sensations of the pulse beating very rapidly or forcefully (called palpitations). The second pointer is that the symptoms are not necessarily related to posture. Symptoms that come on while sitting down are much more likely to be arrhythmias, and if they come on lying flat then the chances are higher still. Abnormal rhythms are much more common in people who already have a history of heart disease.

◆ **Atrial fibrillation** is a chaotic irregular heart rhythm which affects about one in seven people over the age of 75. It is not uncommon for the heart beat suddenly to speed up, particularly in response to an infection or any other illness. People who normally have a regular heart beat can suddenly develop episodes of atrial fibrillation, which can last from a few seconds to a few days. When the heart's rhythm suddenly becomes irregular there is a significant drop in the amount of blood pumped by the heart, with a drop in the blood pressure which may be sufficient to cause fainting.

◆ **Supraventricular tachycardia** is similar, although the heart beat remains regular throughout. Patients often have a long history of episodes, perhaps going back into their youth. In other cases it is associated with illness, and particularly with heart disease.

◆ **Ventricular tachycardia** is a much more serious type of irregular abnormal rapid heart beat. The normal mechanism by which electrical impulses are conducted from the top to the bottom of the heart is not used. The electrical stimulus causing the heart to contract originates in the ventricles, the lower part of the heart. This results in inefficient contraction, reduced output, and a risk of inadequate heart activity to sustain life. Because of the inadequate pumping activity and reduced output, ventricular tachycardia often gives rise to giddiness or fainting. Ventricular tachycardia is a serious and potentially life-threatening condition. It can degenerate to ventricular fibrillation, which is usually fatal.

Sick sinus syndrome

There are several conditions in which the heart rate is too slow. The most common of these is **sick sinus syndrome**, a thickening of the conducting tissues with age. This leads to periods in which the heart pauses for a few seconds, and other periods when it sets up abnormally rapid rhythms such as rapid atrial fibrillation. The treatment of this condition is with a pacemaker together with medication to slow the heart down.

Heart block occurs when the normal mechanism of conduction of electrical impulses in the heart is blocked through damage to the conducting tissues. This usually occurs as a consequence of heart attacks, angina, or aortic valve disease, or simply with thickening of the tissues with advancing age.

There are several forms of heart block, but in complete heart block, the most severe form, the heart typically slows down to about 30 beats/min, resulting in symptoms of giddiness or possibly passing out. The only effective treatment is with a pacemaker.

In some patients the normal mechanisms of conduction may continue to work properly, but an impulse is set off too infrequently to maintain proper output from the heart. The heart beats regularly, but only at a rate of 30–50 beats/min. This also requires treatment with a pacemaker.

Detecting abnormal heart rhythms

Abnormal heart rhythms are common. A third of normal people over 75 have them intermittently, and they are the same rhythms as are found in people who are falling and passing out. It is very difficult to establish when these rhythms are really the cause of the symptoms unless a recording can be obtained at the time when symptoms occur. Many people have these symptoms very infrequently, perhaps once or twice a year, and so it is unlikely that they will be detected by a 24-hour recording of the heart rhythm.

An abnormal heart rhythm may be detected on a routine ECG. Usually, longer periods of ECG recording are needed, and require an external ECG recorder which is worn for periods of between 24 hours and 2 weeks. If that is insufficient, a device called a Reveal, which is about the size of a little finger, is put in under the skin above the breast. This can record abnormal rhythms for up to 18 months. It is helpful in some difficult cases, but requires a minor operation to insert it and to remove it.

In many patients who have recurrent episodes of loss of consciousness a pacemaker is inserted without a clear diagnosis of the abnormal rhythm. In about half of such cases the patient continues to pass out because the irregular rhythm is not the cause of their unconsciousness.

📄 Case history

Helen was an 83-year-old woman who had been admitted to hospital three times in the previous 4 weeks. On each occasion she had experienced chest pains and shortness of breath. She had also had a few episodes where she fell without explanation.

On this occasion the cause for her falls was obvious. Her ECG showed a period of heart block, which subsequently returned to a normal rhythm. She was listed for a pacemaker.

While on the ward waiting for this, she suddenly became confused, short of breath, and started to complain of chest pain. These were the symptoms that had caused her four admissions, for which no cause had been found.

Her blood pressure had dropped from 160/80 to 110/70 mmHg, and her pulse had become rapid and irregular. An ECG showed that she had gone into rapid atrial fibrillation at a rate of 150 beats/min. At this rate, her heart was not filling adequately with blood at each beat, causing a reduction in the amount of blood pumped around the circulation. Her confusion was due to the sudden reduction in blood flow to the brain.

Her symptoms were controlled with a beta-blocker, and a pacemaker was put in. After that she remained completely well, with no more falls.

Non-cardiac causes of loss of consciousness

There are other causes of unconsciousness, but they usually present differently. There is one important situation in which confusion can arise.

A sudden reduction in blood supply to the brain can cause fits (termed secondary seizures). Whereas cardiac syncope causes only brief unconsciousness, that caused by fits is usually more prolonged.

If there is such a fit as a result of diminished blood flow to the brain, the history sounds like that of a fit, not of syncope. Such patients are commonly misdiagnosed as having epilepsy, with all the restrictions that then apply. They will be barred from driving and may lose their jobs. If they have recurrent syncope, they will be labelled as having epilepsy unresponsive to treatment, and find themselves taking more and more tablets for their non-existent epilepsy. Proving that the diagnosis is syncope (usually through tilt-table testing) is very helpful.

Most other causes produce longer periods of unconsciousness, and this is usually evident from the history. Only occasionally are such patients referred because they are reported to have had a fall.

10

Medicines and falls

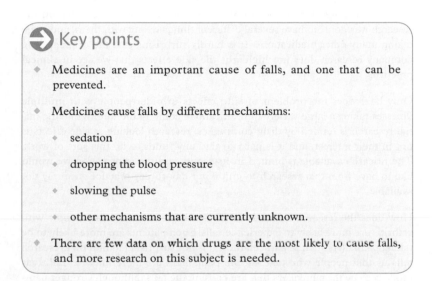

Key points

- Medicines are an important cause of falls, and one that can be prevented.

- Medicines cause falls by different mechanisms:

  - sedation

  - dropping the blood pressure

  - slowing the pulse

  - other mechanisms that are currently unknown.

- There are few data on which drugs are the most likely to cause falls, and more research on this subject is needed.

In a significant minority of falls medicines may be the cause, or one among several causes, of falls. Most medicines do not cause falls.

Although there is no doubt that some medicines can cause falls, the *British National Formulary* (the book that doctors use to check on drug doses and side effects) does not include falls as a side effect for any medication. The problem is to decide which medicines are the ones responsible, and to find an alternative that will have the necessary therapeutic effects but not have the same side effects.

The research that has been has been done in this field gives us only limited information, some of which is misleading. Most drug research is focused on new drugs, and on what their potential benefits might be. Little information is available from research that is designed to look at the problem of side effects. Falls become a problem from the age of 75 onwards, and few research projects contain many patients aged over 75. Research to show the benefits of new medicines is usually carried out in people who are middle-aged, and have only the condition that is being studied. Such people are usually taking few, if any, other medicines. Their ability to get themselves to a clinic for follow-up implies that they are otherwise fit and mobile.

Once the research establishing the benefit of a drug is published, it starts to be used more frequently in anyone who has the condition in question. These people are likely to be about 20 years older than those in whom the research was done, to have several different things wrong with them, and to be taking many other medications. It is hardly surprising that the original drug company research does not highlight the side effects that we see in clinical practice.

Only later does the problem of side effects in older people with multiple illnesses taking a large variety of medications come to the fore. While the initial research is funded by drug companies, research looking at side effects is not in their interest, and it is hard to find any funds to do this sort of work. The research available is limited in its scope, and the information we would like to have from that research to guide our day-to-day practice is simply not available.

How does the research mislead us? For example, we know that people with arthritis are more likely to experience falls. Such patients are more likely to be taking painkillers such as paracetamol. It is not surprising to find that research tells us that people who take simple painkillers are more likely to fall. It is unlikely to be the painkillers that are causing the falls (although stronger pain-killers containing codeine or morphine might do so).

People who take more than four types of medicine have an increased risk of falling. Most types of medicine do not contribute to falling, but the more medicines you take, the more likely it is that one of them may be do so. The more medicines you take, the more likely it is that you have multiple problems, some of which may make you more likely to fall. It is hard to think of five types of different medicines that can be given without the fifth being of a type that might predispose to falls.

If you have fallen, and are taking any of the following medications:

◆ for high blood pressure

◆ for diabetes

◆ for angina

◆ for heart disease

◆ strong painkillers

◆ for depression

◆ for anxiety

◆ sleeping tablets

◆ for an enlarged prostate

you should consult your doctor, because your tablets may be responsible for your falls, or may be contributing to them.

People with anxiety and depression are also prone to falling. Sedatives and antidepressants are strongly related to an increased risk of falling, but in this case it is probable that the medications are to blame because they slow reaction times. Two types of antidepressant are in common use. Tricyclics are the older group, and are poorly tolerated because of their side effects. They cause sedation and orthostatic hypotension. We might expect these tablets to cause falls. Selective serotonin-reuptake inhibitors (SSRIs) rarely cause orthostatic hypotension and are not sedating. However, research shows that, for reasons that are unclear, one group is as bad as the other in terms of falls risk.

As people grow older, there is a tendency for them to tolerate medicines less well. They may be more sensitive to the effects of the drugs, and need lower doses. This is particularly true of sleeping tablets. They are also likely to have more frequent side effects, and ones that are more serious. They are unable to get the drug out of their system as well as the younger people do (because of reduced activity in the liver and the kidney, which the body uses to eliminate most medicines).

Older people usually have less muscle and water, and more fat, in their bodies than younger people, and this affects the way in which medicines are distributed within the body, usually resulting in higher effective drug levels than in younger people.

It is not always possible to stop medicines that are contributing to falling. It may be that without them the patient would be much worse off, and at risk of becoming seriously ill. Some patients take large amounts of strong painkilling medications which cause falls. Faced with a choice of falling, or having their pain, they will often choose to continue the medication. Sometimes an alternative treatment that has the same benefits but fewer side effects can be found. Sometimes all that is needed is a reduction in the dose.

However, there are occasions when stopping the drug is not a realistic option. In one study, there was a dramatic reduction in falls when patients in a nursing home had all their sedatives and sleeping tablets stopped. Within a few weeks of the study finishing, most of the patients had been restarted on their previous medication.

Many patients take more than one medicine that is commonly associated with falling. Trying to establish which particular medicine is the one that is causing their falls is difficult. The medicines are usually ones that they need. They may be unwell if they are stopped. There may be no safer equivalent available. Trying to sort out such cases is time consuming and difficult, as it is hard to know whether the medicines really are the cause of the falls, which medicines to stop, and what to replace them with.

There are several different mechanisms whereby medicines can cause falls. The main ones are:

◆ lowering the blood pressure

◆ slowing the pulse rate

◆ reducing the volume of blood in the circulation, which reduces the blood pressure

◆ slowing the mental processes of the brain, dulling the senses and increasing reaction times.

Some medicines have more than one effect that can contribute to falling.

Lowering blood pressure

Treatments that lower blood pressure given for conditions other than high blood pressure

Logically one would expect medication that reduces blood pressure to be given only to those whose blood pressure is raised. A high blood pressure is found in about half of people over the age of 75 (exactly what proportion depends on how you define high blood pressure). However, many people who take medication that reduces blood pressure have a normal blood pressure to start with, or even one that is low. There are a considerable number of conditions other than having high blood pressure for which blood-pressure-lowering medication is prescribed. Not surprisingly, a proportion of people are unable to tolerate the reduction in blood pressure to below-normal levels caused by their medication, and many of them develop giddiness, falls, or faints.

The reasons that blood-pressure-reducing medications are used for the above conditions fall into two main categories.

In some cases the medication used has several different effects: the one desired for the condition being treated, but also a reduction in blood pressure as an unwanted effect. For example, doxazosin and prazosin, which are used to open up the urethra (the tube from the bladder to the penis) in men with an enlarged prostate, making it easier to pass urine, are also very potent blood pressure medicines and tend to cause severe orthostatic hypotension. These drugs have been largely superseded by more modern agents (tamsulosin, alfluzosin) which have an effect on the urethra, but are said to have less effect on blood pressure.

A class of drugs called beta-blockers has numerous effects, one of which is to reduce blood pressure. Beta-blockers are used to treat angina, to improve life expectancy after heart attacks and in heart failure, to treat anxiety, to treat over-active thyroid glands, and to treat shaking of the limbs (essential tremor). They are also used as eye drops for glaucoma. People who take beta-blockers may suffer from drops in their blood pressure sufficient to cause symptoms. They may also find that their pulse rate has slowed so that there is insufficient blood flow to the brain.

The other reason that blood-pressure-reducing medications are used is to reduce the blood pressure to a level as low as can be tolerated. Any hydraulic system will last longer, and be less likely to spring a leak, if it is run at a lower pressure. This is as true of the circulation as it is of domestic plumbing. This strategy is used to increase life expectancy in people who have diabetes, kidney failure, heart failure, and stroke. The aim is to reduce the blood pressure to the lowest level that the patient can tolerate. Following stroke, for example, your chances of having another stroke are diminished by reducing the blood pressure, and the more the blood pressure is reduced (with no lower limit), the lower the risk of another stroke. Thus there is a great temptation to reduce the blood pressure to levels that lead to faintness and falls.

High blood pressure

Medicines used to treat high blood pressure all have the potential to reduce blood pressure to levels that cause faintness. Treating high blood pressure involves getting the right balance for each individual, and what suits one person may not suit another.

Although your doctor can check whether your medication is lowering your blood pressure to very low levels, that is not the point. These medications produce their adverse side effects in general by allowing brief sudden drops in blood pressure (see Chapter 7), and not by keeping the blood pressure low all the time.

Slowing the pulse rate

Drugs used to regulate the heart rate:

- beta-blockers

- digoxin

- calcium-channel blockers: verapamil, diltiazem

- amiodarone.

There are several conditions in which it is useful to slow the pulse rate. Most commonly this is when the pulse is irregular or has a tendency to race—rapid atrial fibrillation and supraventricular tachycardia. However, drugs that slow the heart rate are also used for other purposes, such as angina and cardiac failure, and then the slowing of the heart rate can be an undesirable side effect.

When the heart rate slows too much—to below 50 beats/min—there is a chance that there will be a fall in blood flow to the brain sufficient to cause giddiness, falls, and syncope.

Case history

Ethel was an 85-year-old woman who had lived with her sister all her life. Upon her sister's death she went into a care home. In her sixties she had developed shaking of her hands whenever she tried to do anything (an essential tremor). This had progressed slowly, so that eventually she had difficulty getting food to her mouth.

The shaking had begun to affect her head and her mouth, and she became distressed by it. Her GP started her on propranolol 40 mg three times a day, which is the standard treatment for this condition, and there was some improvement in her shaking.

After about 3 years on this medication she was referred to a falls specialist because she had fallen without warning on about 12 occasions. She denied ever losing consciousness, and said that she never experienced giddiness.

She was found to have a pulse rate of 45 beats/min (normal is about 80 beats/min, and less than 50 beats/min is significantly slow). Her blood pressure was low, at 110/70 mmHg when lying, and fell further to 90/60 mmHg on standing.

The propranolol was stopped, and she was started on primidone, which she found to be more effective in controlling her symptoms. She stopped falling. Her pulse rate and blood pressure both returned to normal.

Reducing the volume of blood in the circulation

Medications that cause an increase in the volume of urine produced are called diuretics. They are used commonly for two conditions—high blood pressure and heart failure. A different type of diuretic is used for each condition.

The type of diuretic used to reduce blood pressure is called a thiazide, and it works primarily by opening up blood vessels. The effect on urine production is rarely commented on by patients, and is not dramatic. Nevertheless, it can be shown that patients who take this type of medication can have a reduced amount of fluid in the circulation, and one study shows that 65 per cent of older patients taking a thiazide had orthostatic hypotension.

A different type of medication, either furosemide or bumetanide, is used for heart failure. This has a much stronger action, which may be sudden and disturbing for the patient. These medications have their effect by increasing the amount of salt the kidneys eliminate, with water being lost with the salt. They can produce severe states of dehydration if taken in excess.

Most commonly patients take these types of diuretics for years, and find themselves in a situation where the medications are producing a tendency to faint that would otherwise not be of a magnitude to cause symptoms. Unfortunately, those who need diuretics for heart failure have no alternative, and such medicines have to be taken for life. The only thing we can do is to adjust the dose, and to look at what other medicines are being taken that are less critical.

Dulling the senses and slowing reaction times

Relieving pain (whether physical or psychological), getting off to sleep, reducing anxiety, and lifting depression may involve treatments that can cause dulling of the senses. Yet these same senses are the ones that we use to maintain an upright posture.

Many medicines work by slowing the working of the brain, or of nerve cells elsewhere. The outcome is a predictable increase in falls among those who take them.

Maintaining balance requires taking all the information coming into the brain about its position in space from nerves, the inner ear, and the eyes, and using it to judge the position in space and adjust the posture to keep balanced. Anything that interferes with this pathway is sure to make balance worse and falls more probable. Sedative medications will slow the response to a change in position, so that the fine movements required to retain balance will be made more slowly and less accurately. They will also slow or prevent the conscious movements that are made to anticipate changes in balance. Most of the time it will not matter, but every now and then this slowness will result in a fall through not responding quickly enough.

Culprit drugs

Most medicines do not have any of the effects listed above, and are unlikely to contribute to falling. Even when people take medicines that have the effects listed above, the degree to which they are contributing to falls is very difficult to assess. Commonly these drugs are stopped, but the falls continue. Because there are so many factors contributing to the risk of falling, finding one that is possibly significant and rectifying it does not guarantee that the problem will be solved.

It would be useful to have a 'league table' of the effects on falling of various medications. Such information is not available, and in any case the effects of any given drug vary considerably from one person to another, as do the side effects. In some cases the medication is well tolerated for many years, but only causes a problem when the patient becomes ill (particularly with an infection or an illness that causes dehydration).

However, there are certain medications which have a predictable effect that is likely to contribute to falling. As prescribing patterns vary so greatly, in terms of which drugs are used and at what dosage, doctors in different parts of the country will see different problems, and the list of 'culprit drugs' applies to what I see in Oxfordshire. Many drugs can cause falls, but most of the drug-related falls that I see are due to one of the medicines described below.

Antidepressants

Tricyclic antidepressants (amitriptyline, dosulepin, imipramine, and others) have been used to treat depression since the 1970s. They are effective, but have many side effects that are troublesome, and overdosage can be fatal. Although they have been largely superseded by newer drugs in the treatment of depression, they are still commonly used for other purposes.

These drugs are sedating and many people use them as sleeping tablets. The sedation can continue into the next day, slowing reaction times and dulling people's sense of balance. They were originally developed by a company trying to develop a treatment for hay fever (an antihistamine), and their antidepressant effect was unexpected. They were the mainstay of treatment for depression for about 20 years until less sedating drugs were developed. They all have an effect on blood vessels that results in reductions in blood pressure and predictable orthostatic hypotension.

Tricyclic antidepressants are also used to numb chronic pain. For many people their effect on relieving pain and giving a good night's sleep is so important that unsteadiness and a tendency to fall is an acceptable price to pay.

The side effects of tricyclic antidepressants and the risk of depressed patients dying after taking an overdose mean that they have largely been superseded.

Mianserin and mirtazapine are related drugs that are very sedating.

Selective serotonin-reuptake inhibitors (SSRIs) have taken over from tricyclics as the most commonly used treatments for depression. They include fluoxetine (Prozac), citalopram, sertraline, and paroxetine.

Uncommonly, these newer drugs can cause dizziness or orthostatic hypotension, but in most cases they do not. They are not usually sedating, but rather give the patient a 'high'. However, studies show that they are as likely as tricyclics to cause falls. This finding has been reported in several independent studies, but the mechanism by which they do this remains unclear.

Selective noradrenaline-reuptake inhibitors (SNRIs) such as venlafaxine are not very sedating, but can cause severe orthostatic hypotension.

Choosing an antidepressant for people who fall or who have orthostatic hypotension is a problem. Moclobemide is an old drug that is known to cause little, if any, orthostatic hypotension, and which is not sedating. Whether it causes falls through the same unknown mechanisms as SSRIs is not known, as it has not been used sufficiently for data to be available. There is little evidence showing that any one antidepressant is better than any other in mild to moderate depression, and this cheap old-fashioned drug appears to be well tolerated.

📋 Case history

Ken was a 77-year-old man who had developed severe depression. He had started an antidepressant called duloxetine, which had improved his depression considerably. About 4 weeks after starting this medication, he had a couple of unexplained falls at home. On his third fall he bumped his head and became unconscious.

He was brought to hospital, where an emergency brain scan showed bleeding around the brain (a subdural haematoma). This was operated on, and his condition improved. At that stage he was transferred to my ward.

I found him to have severe orthostatic hypotension, with a blood pressure that fell from 160/90 mmHg when lying to 80/50 mmHg on standing. He then had two further falls on the ward, and broke his right hip during the second one. This required an operation.

After that his duloxetine was stopped. His blood pressure improved, and he had only a small drop on standing with no giddiness. He made a good recovery, and went home. A decision was taken to treat any further episodes of depression with moclobemide, an antidepressant that does not cause significant orthostatic hypotension.

Alpha-receptor blockers

Alpha-receptor blockers (doxazosin, prazosin, indoramin) are primarily used to treat high blood pressure. They have been largely superseded by newer drugs, and tend to be reserved for patients who do not respond to other medicines. They are also used for men who have an enlarged prostate and have difficulty passing urine. They commonly cause orthostatic hypotension, and are poorly tolerated in older people.

Sleeping tablets and other sedatives

Sleeping tablets are supposed to get you off to sleep, and then to be out of your system by the morning. However, there are two problems.

Firstly, many elderly people have to get up at night to go to the toilet. The sleeping tablet is still working on them, and they get up in a drugged state. As a result their balance is impaired, their reflexes are slowed, and their risk of falling is very high.

The second problem is that the drug is often not out of their system by the morning. The sedative effects can continue well into the next day. The way in which these drugs are eliminated or broken down by the body is often less effective in older people, and the brain is more sensitive to their effects. A dose that would be too small to be effective for a middle-aged person might be dangerously high for someone who is older.

As people grow older, they need less sleep but their day is less full of activity. They may have slept 7 or 8 hours every day throughout their adult lives, but can now only sleep for 4 or 5 hours at night, with naps in the afternoon. They try to restore a normal adult sleeping pattern by use of sleeping tablets. Frustration that this does not work may lead to increasing dosages and dependency on the sleeping tablets.

ACE inhibitors

Angiotensin-converting enzyme (ACE) inhibitors are prescribed very frequently. Although most people tolerate them very well, because they are used so much, the small proportion of people who do not tolerate them reaches a significant number.

One major problem with these medicines is the desire to achieve the highest possible dose to obtain the greatest benefit. Many older people do not tolerate these higher doses.

They are used increasingly in the treatment of high blood pressure. In some people they may cause orthostatic hypotension or vasovagal syndrome. One study looking at older people taking such a drug, in this case lisinopril, found that 60 per cent of them had orthostatic hypotension. The side effects are usually dependent upon the dose.

They are used frequently in people whose blood pressure is normal or low to start with (i.e. for conditions other than high blood pressure). It is hardly surprising that this should cause falls or faintness in some people when their blood pressure is reduced too much.

A related class of drug, angiotensin-receptor blockers (ARBs), have all the benefits of angiotensin converting enzyme inhibitors, but may have fewer side effects. There is little research in this field, but in clinical practice these newer drugs appear to have much less effect on blood pressure control.

Beta-blockers

Beta-blockers are well-established drugs that have many uses, and they have an excellent safety record. However, they have predictable side effects in a small number of people, or if the dose is too high.

They can cause the pulse to become too slow, and can make sick sinus syndrome and carotid sinus hypersensitivity worse. They always cause some reduction in the pulse rate, but this gives rise to symptoms in only a small proportion of cases. Some people take beta-blockers for many years, and then suddenly develop a problem with their pulse. This probably reflects the way in which the ageing process makes the heart's conducting system more sensitive to these adverse effects.

Beta-blockers are also used as eye drops to treat glaucoma. Even then, they are absorbed in sufficient amounts to affect the heart.

11

Confusion, poor memory, and falls

> ## ➜ Key points
>
> ◆ Forgetfulness is a normal part of ageing.
>
> ◆ Dementia is a disease process which results in impairment of thought processes and memory, particularly short-term memory.
>
> ◆ Delirium (acute confusion) is a short-term state of confusion and agitation, usually as the result of some illness.
>
> ◆ The risk of falls increases dramatically when confused people find themselves in a new environment. The risk diminishes gradually over a number of weeks.
>
> ◆ The combination of confusion, long-standing ill health, and a minor illness leading to a fall is a common reason for admission to hospital.

As people grow older, so their memory deteriorates, particularly that for recent events, i.e. the short-term memory. Distant events are remembered better than recent ones, and people focus more and more on things that happened years ago. This absent-mindedness is a normal part of the ageing process, but in some people there is a deterioration in mental function that goes beyond forgetfulness.

Dementia

Dementia is said to occur when the brain's thought processes are affected by wearing out of the brain's ability to function. This is not just a gradual decline in the activity of cells in the brain, but the result of disease processes, often resulting in abnormal proteins which interfere with brain function being produced and deposited within the brain substance. The most common, and the best known, of the dementias is Alzheimer's disease, named after Alois Alzheimer, the German doctor who first described it in 1911.

Alzheimer's disease is common in older people and, with the rapid increase in the number of very old people, is now one of the greatest challenges to health systems in the developed world. About 20 per cent of people over the age of 80 years in the UK have some evidence of dementia. A larger percentage have some early impairment of thought processes and memory (termed cognitive impairment), which may or may not progress to dementia.

Delirium

The term delirium or 'acute confusional state' is used for people who become very muddled, and often agitated as a result of something that has upset their system either suddenly or over a number of days (or even a few weeks). This is usually the result of an illnes—almost any illness, but most commonly an infection—or the side effects of medication. Patients with delirium may already suffer from dementia, with a marked worsening of their confusion and agitation. However, many have no evidence of dementia and make a full recovery from their delirium.

Impaired memory and thought are common in other illnesses, particularly in those people who have had previous strokes, and in Parkinson's disease and related conditions.

Many patients with these conditions will not be very strong or fit, and the loss of muscle strength and physical capability, together with the specific problems of weakness or stiffness caused by their illness, will make them very prone to falling. Any illness, even a minor infection, will make this much worse, as well as making them more muddled. People in this group—the infected patients with poor physical health and delirium or dementia—are those who are the most likely to fall among all of the patients I see. Any hospital emergency department will see patients like this every day.

Confusion and falls

Staying upright involves making a large number of decisions that allow you to do things safely: where to put your feet, what to hold on to, where and when to sit down. People with cognitive impairment lose the ability to make these judgements properly and consistently. They find it difficult to make movements which anticipate changes in balance reliably. When they make an error of judgement, they may do something that makes them likely to fall.

Balance is challenged when attention is diverted to another task. People with dementia are particularly affected by this, as they have smaller reserves of brain function to distribute between these tasks, and difficulty in switching their attention from one task to another. This impaired mental capacity is usually accompanied by a lack of insight into the problem—there is no problem, as far as the patient is concerned. Their risk of falls is often increased by other factors, such as poor vision and bladder problems causing frequent or urgent use of the toilet.

Things are made much worse when the patient is put in an unfamiliar place, for example a hospital ward or a care home. They do not know where they want to go, perhaps they cannot see to get there, and they are faced with unknown obstacles. Understandably, this makes them anxious. When people move into care homes, it is common for them to fall. Most falls occur in the first few weeks in the home, as they adjust to the new surroundings and become familiar with them. It also takes some time for the staff to get to know them.

Many patients with dementia lose their sense of smell, and this makes them unable to taste food normally. Together with a loss of interest in food, and a tendency to forget to ensure that they have any available, this results in a loss of weight. As a result they become weak and unsteady.

Other people with dementia lose interest in walking. They will do so only when prompted. Naturally they become weak and 'deconditioned' as a result, and when they do try to get up and walk they will be more likely to fall.

What can be done about falls in patients with confusion?

Because of their impaired memory people with dementia may not be able to take in or remember the types of strategy that are used by other fallers. They cannot learn new safer behaviours. They forget to use a stick or a frame. They do not remember to do exercises. This makes organizing help for them very problematic.

A first step should be to review their list of medications; many will be taking medicines that are likely to reduce their blood pressure or slow their reflexes (all sedatives and antidepressants, and some painkillers, can do this). Most such patients take some medications of these types, although sometimes they are essential and cannot be stopped.

The next step is to discuss safe behaviour, the risks of falling, and how to manage them with those who live with or supervise the patient. They may be able to encourage the use of a walking aid, which might make walking safer. Ensuring that they use their glasses, that they have appropriate footwear, and that their feet are well looked after can all help diminish falls risk.

Steps need to be taken to ensure a safe environment for the patient—the removal of hazards, the provision of rails, raised toilet seats, and an alarm system. An appropriate system of care, whether from relatives or from paid carers, needs to be set up to ensure adequate supervision.

In the end, no-one can be made entirely risk free, and as long as all reasonable steps have been taken to ensure safety, some degree of risk has to be allowed. The patients may not agree to much (or any) of this, and often considerable family pressure is required to do everything possible to reduce risk. People with confusion and a history of falls living on their own are a cause of major concern to their families, and it is this group who most frequently have to give up their homes to go into a care home.

People with dementia or delirium have a greatly increased risk of falls.

◆ They have difficulty in making safe judgements reliably about movements to maintain position and balance.

◆ They are often frail, weak, and malnourished.

◆ They frequently take medications that might predispose to falls.

◆ Frequently they cannot learn safe behaviour because of their memory loss.

◆ Their environment needs to be made as safe as possible.

◆ Appropriate systems of care and supervision need to be put in place to help them.

◆ The combination of confusion and falls is the most common reason for needing to go into a care home.

12

Visual problems that can contribute to falls

> ➔ **Key points**
>
> Having the wrong prescription spectacles is the most common visual problem leading to falls.
>
> Eye diseases can lead to impaired vision, and are a major cause of falls.
>
> ◆ Cataracts can only be treated by surgery.
>
> ◆ Macular degeneration is a progressive disorder, for which there is usually no effective treatment.
>
> ◆ Glaucoma is treated with eye drops to prevent an increase in the pressure in the eye.
>
> ◆ Diabetes has several different effects on the eye. Maintaining good diabetic control slows the progression of diabetic eye disease. New vessels are managed with laser treatment.

Spectacles

Impaired vision is a major contributory factor for many people who fall. The most common problems are simple short-sightedness, often since youth, or the long-sightedness that occurs once the lens starts to harden after the age of 40. These problems are corrected with glasses. Many people make do with glasses that do not correct their poor vision well enough.

Glasses often have to correct for both short-sightedness and long-sightedness. Anyone who wears such glasses (bifocals or varifocals) will be aware of the distortion that occurs in the area where the two different strengths of lens meet.

This is in the lower and side parts of the lens, which are used when looking down or to the side. There is some evidence that this distortion is important in judging distance, and may contribute to trips. People who wear such glasses are more likely to catch their foot on a step or kerb by misjudging its height than when they are wearing a single prescription lens.

Poor lighting

Changes in the eye and the brain mean that having the correct amount of light available becomes more important with increasing age. This is particularly important in areas that are hazardous, such as stairs, and areas in which falls tend to occur, such as the bathroom and toilet. In particular, the route to the toilet at night needs to be well lit. The stairs need to be lit brightly enough to be able to recognize where one step ends and the next begins.

Eye diseases

There are four diseases of the eye that are common in the elderly but are seen only rarely in younger people. Between them they account for the overwhelming majority of visual problems in the older age group. In addition, there are several other conditions of the eye that impair vision, which become increasingly common with increasing age. These include blocked blood vessels (venous occlusion), and retinal detachment.

There are four common diseases that affect the eye in later life and can lead to impaired vision:

- cataract

- macular degeneration

- glaucoma

- the effects of diabetes on the eye.

Cataracts develop over a number of years, causing misting of vision and eventually blindness. A cataract is a change in the composition of the lens, causing it to become opaque and to distort and obscure the light passing through it. About a third of people over the age of 65 have a cataract of one or both eyes.

The only treatment for cataracts is an operation to remove the affected lens and insert a false one. The operation is quick and simple, and good vision is restored by the next day.

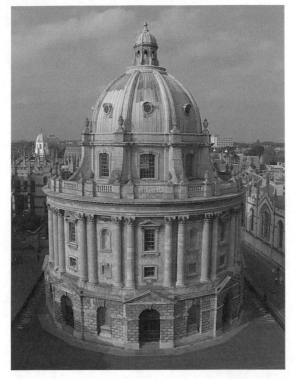

Figure 12.1 Normal vision.

The lens of the eye is normally clear, but with increasing age the material of the lens changes and does not let the light through normally. The image focused on the retina becomes blurred. The mechanisms causing cataracts are poorly understood.

Symptoms of cataract include:

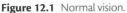

- worsening of vision

- spots in the vision

- glare and haloes from the sun or lights, particularly affecting driving at night

- double vision

- difficulty in distinguishing colours

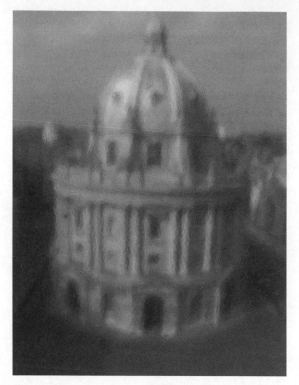

Figure 12.2 Cataract.

◆ frequent changes in prescription glasses as eyesight deteriorates

◆ a temporary initial improvement in near vision as the lens changes shape, which then becomes worse again (called second sight).

📄 Case history

Jane was a 79-year-old woman who lived alone, and had cataracts. She had fallen twice in the house, and was now afraid to walk outside, having previously been active. She felt giddy and unsteady on getting up, and had lost confidence. She was supported at home by two daughters, but was requiring more help than they could manage. The possibility of moving into a care home was being explored.

She had a cataract operation. The next day, she said that she felt dramatically different. The giddiness had gone and she was no longer unsteady. Over the following weeks she got back to her previous level of independence, and was able to walk to the shops on her own. By the time she attended the falls clinic she was a new woman. Such responses are rare, but gratifying for those involved.

As an aside, when she came back to the clinic a few months later she reported that she had had a fall. When she was younger she had worked as an operating theatre sister, but had had to give up because of narcolepsy, an uncontrollable tendency to fall asleep suddenly. Another feature of the narcolepsy syndrome is cataplexy—a sudden loss of strength in all the muscles of the body, often brought on by emotion (and possibly the root of the expression 'to fall down laughing'). Her grandson had bought a billiard table, and invited her to have a go. With her first shot, she potted a ball, and overcome by emotion, promptly collapsed to the floor with an attack of cataplexy. This is a rather unusual cause for a fall.

Macular degeneration is a slow deterioration of the central part of the visual field. The retina is a layer of light-sensitive nerve cells at the back of the eye. When you look at something directly, the information from that object is focused onto the macula, the middle part of the retina. In macular degeneration the middle part of the area of vision becomes obscured and is eventually lost.

Macular degeneration is of two types. The usual type is called 'dry' macular degeneration. The macula seems to dry up and become thinner as nerve cells are lost. There is no effective treatment for 'dry' macular degeneration.

Less commonly, there is increased fluid around the macula, which is termed 'wet' macular degeneration. This form responds to laser treatment to some extent. There are also new medications that slow the progression of this type of macular degeneration.

Glaucoma is a condition in which the pressure of fluid inside the eye increases, leading to damage to the blood vessels entering the eye at the back. This causes the nerve cells in the retina to die off, starting with those at the edge. There is a loss of peripheral vision, which may go unnoticed until it is very advanced. Eventually this leads to loss of all but the central part of vision, and the patient feels as though they are looking at everything through a tunnel. Successful treatment depends on early diagnosis. Once the diagnosis is made, the condition

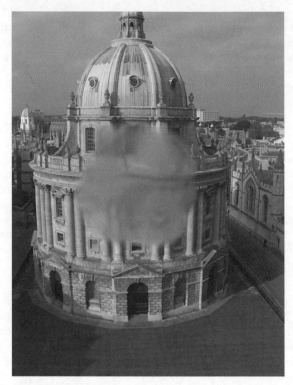

Figure 12.3 Macular degeneration.

can be kept at bay with eye drops, but the damage that has already occurred cannot be reversed.

There is a condition called acute (meaning sudden) glaucoma, in which the eye becomes red and painful, with impairment or loss of vision. This is caused by a sudden increase in eye pressure, and responds to treatment. Most commonly, a small hole is made in the iris (the coloured portion of the eye), which then allows free movement of fluid between the front and the back of the eye.

Diabetes commonly affects the eyes. It is a disease in which all the blood vessels are damaged, and this damage to the vessels leads to an impaired blood supply to various parts of the body. The heart, brain, and kidneys are the organs that suffer most, but the eye tends to be affected to a similar extent.

Diabetes causes an increase in cataracts and glaucoma, but the most damaging condition is diabetic retinopathy (damage to the retina). Damage to the blood vessels causes them to start to leak in the area of the macula, causing a deterioration in central vision. It also results in a lack of oxygen supply to the retina. New blood vessels are produced to overcome this, but these vessels are abnormal. They become a problem because of a tendency to bleed and cause scarring. The treatment is to destroy the new blood vessels with a laser.

13

How does neurological disease cause falls?

→ Key points

Neurological diseases commonly cause falls, and are often the first thing that leads to a medical opinion.

Stroke can cause falls because of:

- muscle weakness
- loss of coordination
- impaired balance
- impaired understanding and judgement.

Parkinson's disease causes falls because of:

- rigidity and stiffness of the muscles, slowing responses
- an abnormal bent posture which threatens stability
- freezing and the inability to complete corrective movements
- loss of the idea of where the vertical lies
- impaired perception of the surrounding space
- diminished cone of stability
- confusion
- orthostatic hypotension.

Epilepsy can cause falls during seizures, or as a side effect of treatment.

Peripheral neuropathies can cause falls because of:

♦ loss of body sensation

♦ weakness

♦ autonomic neuropathy causing orthostatic hypotension.

Standing up is entirely dependent on the nervous system functioning properly, and anything that affects the nervous system can interfere with sensation, balance, coordination, and muscle strength. The nervous control of blood pressure is also affected in several diseases.

It is common in a falls clinic for a patient with an undiagnosed neurological condition to be referred because of falls. The fall may be the first symptom of an illness which may well progress steadily, or which may respond to treatment. Rapid and accurate diagnosis is important. We regularly diagnose new cases of stroke, Parkinson's disease, and epilepsy in patients who did not suspect that there was a more significant underlying illness causing their falls.

A fall may be the first symptom of an underlying neurological disease.

Stroke

Stroke is a condition in which part of the brain is damaged by problems with its blood supply.

The word 'stroke' comes from a medieval English expression 'the stroke of the hand of God', which is very appropriate, as a stroke comes on suddenly and without warning.

The familiar type of stroke is that which causes paralysis down one side. This tends to recover partially over a period of weeks or months, but there is frequently some residual loss of strength and balance. The greatest risk of falling occurs during the recovery period, when the patient is encouraged to do more and more for him- or herself, and has to take risks in order to make progress.

The type of stroke in which one side is paralysed is the tip of an iceberg of stroke disease. Many strokes have only minor or brief symptoms, and strength, balance, and coordination can be affected in many different ways. Strokes in the back part of the brain (the brainstem and cerebellum) will specifically damage areas involved in the control of balance.

There are several different mechanisms that can cause a stroke.

◆ Most commonly, a clot forms within the blood vessels of the head and neck, or in the heart, and shoots off causing blockage of a vessel downstream. The tissue that gets its blood supply from that vessel dies, and the functions of that part of the brain are lost.

◆ Some strokes are due to blood vessels bursting, causing bleeding into the brain tissue and local damage. Sometimes this is the consequence of that part of the brain being damaged by a clot, as above.

◆ Other strokes are due to a small blood vessel clotting off spontaneously.

In some people there are no clear episodes of stroke symptoms, but a gradual process of damage to tiny vessels that has a cumulative effect. This is called 'small vessel disease'.

After a stroke there are a number of things that can predispose to falls.

◆ The sense of balance may be affected in such a way that standing or walking is difficult without support.

◆ Weakness down one side may leave the patient unable to generate enough force in the affected leg to stand upon it reliably.

◆ The weakness may prevent the affected leg from being swung through effectively during walking.

◆ In particular, if the muscles holding the foot up are weak, the foot may catch on the floor causing a trip.

◆ Walking is slower.

◆ The gait may be abnormal in a variety of ways depending on the site and severity of the stroke.

◆ The patient's idea of the surrounding world can be altered by stroke when it causes a tendency to neglect one side (sensory neglect or sensory inattention).

◆ There may be visual loss to one side as a result of damage to visual pathways within the brain (hemianopia).

◆ The sense of vertical may be distorted because of damage to those parts of the brain in which the body's sensations are interpreted. This can result in inappropriate movements while attempting to rebalance, when the patient moves towards what they think is upright, but makes a movement that adds to their instability.

◆ There may be a lack of understanding of where the limits of stability are (see Chapter 2), and these may be misrepresented or misunderstood by the damaged brain.

Transient ischaemic attack

A small stroke whose symptoms have gone away completely within 24 hours is called a transient ischaemic attack (TIA). It is a minor stroke, and there is often some permanent damage to the brain tissue, although this is usually small. TIAs need urgent investigation and treatment, as there is a significant risk of further strokes which is highest in the first 2 weeks.

A fall may be the main symptom of a transient ischaemic attack, and in our falls clinic TIAs are a common cause for referral. Recurrent falls or recurrent episodes of loss of consciousness are virtually never due to TIAs.

Small vessel disease

Small vessel disease involves large numbers of tiny strokes throughout the brain, which have a cumulative effect. It occurs particularly in people who are smokers, or who have high blood pressure or diabetes. The most common symptoms are difficulty in walking and postural giddiness.

The effect of small vessel disease of the brain is very important. It is extremely common with increasing age (one might say that minor degrees are normal). It disrupts pathways that join all the different parts of the brain. Often this is not to a degree that causes obvious symptoms or signs that can be found on examination. It simply slows the working of the nervous system, leading to forgetfulness, unsteadiness, dizziness, bladder problems, physical slowing, and a multitude of other things that we put down to just growing older. Characteristically, patients with more advanced small vessel disease walk slowly with small steps. They may have great difficulty in turning, and seem not to know what to do with their feet, which often look as though they are stuck to the ground.

Small vessel disease can lead to generalized stiffness of the muscles, a condition that can resemble Parkinson's disease. It can also cause progressive memory loss (or in extreme cases a 'vascular dementia').

Parkinson's disease

> Parkinson's disease is a slowly progressive condition caused by a gradual deterioration of a small part of the brain called the substantia nigra (Latin for 'black substance') in which the transmitter substance dopamine is produced. It is the lack of dopamine (and other substances) in the brain which leads to the symptoms of Parkinson's disease. This area of the brain is black because of a high concentration of a substance called neuromelanin.

The characteristic symptom of Parkinson's disease is shaking of the arms, which is rhythmic at 5 cycles per second, worse at rest, and better when using the arm. More commonly, however, in later life the disease presents with increased stiffness of the limbs and a generalized slowing of movement (rigidity and 'bradykinesia' (Greek for 'slow movement')). It also causes difficulty with balance, and a tendency to fall. Early symptoms are difficulty in turning over in bed at night, a reduced ability to walk at speed or for any great distance, a deterioration in writing, which usually becomes smaller, and difficulty with fine movements, such as doing up buttons.

Falls in Parkinson's disease are complex:

- the ability to sense that balance has been lost is impaired

- the ability to make rapid accurate corrective movements has also gone

- there is a tendency to freeze

- movements are initiated that cannot be completed, but cause loss of balance

- patients have a disordered idea of the space around them.

- patients lose the idea of where vertical lies, and make adjustments to their position that fail to restore balance

- the cone of stability is greatly diminished (see Chapter 2).

Parkinson's disease causes the patient to have a bent posture, looking down at the ground. Bending in this way moves the centre of gravity of the body further forward, so that it is over the front of the feet. Thus the patient cannot walk normally, and takes short shuffling steps to allow his feet to catch up with his centre of gravity.

Falls are common in Parkinson's disease, and injuries commonly result. In one survey, 13 per cent of patients with Parkinson's disease reported falling at least once a week. While most people fall with their legs crumpling beneath them, patients with Parkinson's disease fall at their full length, increasing the risk of injury.

The other problem that commonly occurs in Parkinson's disease is orthostatic hypotension. Partly this is because these patients are of an age where orthostatic hypotension and the other illnesses (and medications) that cause it are common. It can also be part of the disease, or a side effect of some of the treatments. Sadly, orthostatic hypotension in Parkinson's disease responds poorly to treatment.

The management of falls in Parkinson's disease involves many things, but in particular making sure that the patient is on the right treatment for the disease. Such treatment regimes are complicated, and they need to be supervised by a doctor with a particular interest in this condition.

The other factors in management are those common to all fallers—a review of medication, a check for orthostatic hypotension, an assessment of walking aids, physiotherapy to strengthen muscles and improve balance, a home assessment, and an education programme about falls.

Parkinsonism and **Parkinsonian syndromes** are terms used for clinical conditions which resemble Parkinson's disease, but are caused by a different process going on in the brain. These patients respond less well to treatment.

Drug-induced Parkinsonism is the consequence of prolonged use of medication to control psychological symptoms. Two types of medication cause these side effects—phenothiazines (chlorpromazine, fluphenazine, and several others) and butyrophenones (haloperidol). Usually these patients have schizophrenia, hallucinations, or related illnesses. In the past depression was treated with these medicines. The first step in managing drug-induced Parkinsonism is to stop the offending medication. Because of the patient's psychological state this is not always possible, but in most cases the drugs can be stopped or substituted with more modern alternatives which do not have the same side effects. A proportion of patients with drug-induced Parkinsonism show some improvement with anti-Parkinsonian medication, and this should be tried.

Parkinsonian syndromes are a group of conditions which resemble Parkinson's disease, but show little or no response to treatment. These include a list of obscure diseases associated with degeneration of some parts of the brain. Some patients with small vessel disease look as though they have Parkinson's disease, as do people with recurrent head injuries.

Cerebellar disease can occur as the result of stroke, excessive alcohol, certain drugs, and a variety of degenerative conditions such as multiple sclerosis. In addition, damage to the areas of the brainstem through which nerve fibres from the cerebellum pass on their way to and from other parts of the brain cause similar symptoms. Patients with cerebellar disease lose their ability to coordinate. This is seen most easily in the arms, but also affects the trunk and the legs. They walk as though they are drunk—staggering, with irregular step lengths. Such patients often refuse to go out of the house because of what others will think of them. They are unstable when walking, and this results in a wide-based gait—they spread their feet apart as they walk to prevent themselves from falling over.

📄 Case history

Jenny was 83. She had been walking unsteadily for the previous year, and had had three falls in 2 months. She had been diagnosed as epileptic at the age of 21, and had been on treatment with phenytoin (epanutin) for most of this time.

Her walking and arm movements were uncoordinated. She had difficulty in touching the tip of her nose with her finger. She walked as though drunk, with her feet wide apart.

Her phenytoin level was three times the target level. She reduced the dose, and her symptoms improved, but did not go away completely.

Taking too much phenytoin can cause symptoms of cerebellar problems. Phenytoin can also cause permanent cerebellar damage when given in high doses for too long.

Epilepsy

Epilepsy is an important diagnosis in people who lose consciousness and fall as a result. It is also a very difficult diagnosis, because any condition that causes loss of consciousness by diminishing the blood supply to the brain can cause a secondary seizure (see Chapter 9), which can create the impression that the problem is epilepsy. Many people who lose consciousness are misdiagnosed as epileptic, and many have treatment in error for decades for poorly controlled epilepsy.

Epilepsy is a tendency to have seizures (also called fits). Seizures are moments of abnormal electrical activity in the brain. They manifest themselves in a large number of different ways, ranging from barely noticeable moments of absence, a few twitching movements, or a brief episode of unconsciousness, to generalized seizures (which used to be called grand mal epilepsy) with a period of rigidity followed by generalized shaking of all four limbs.

Epilepsy as a cause of unexplained falls is not common, but it does happen. It is difficult to diagnose in the absence of a witness account. Where it is associated with loss of consciousness, this may be for longer than the brief unconsciousness (a few seconds) that occurs with cardiac or blood pressure problems.

The medications for epilepsy are a further problem, in that they dull the senses and make people more likely to fall. Some of them cause loss of balance as a side effect when the dose is too high. Some can cause permanent loss of balance by damaging the cerebellum (the part of the brain that is particularly concerned with maintaining balance).

Peripheral neuropathies

Peripheral neuropathies are conditions which cause the nerves to the limbs to stop working or to die back. They usually only cause numbness and tingling in the feet and hands. In a minority of cases they progress to cause lack of proprioception (information about position in space) and can cause balance problems. They may cause muscular weakness and immobility if they become severe.

A particular type of neuropathy that affects the blood pressure mechanism is an autonomic neuropathy. The autonomic nervous system provides the nerve supply to the gut, the bladder, and the blood vessels. Damage to it is common in vitamin B_{12} deficiency and in long-standing diabetes, but also occurs in other rare conditions. It is believed that the autonomic nerves degenerate with age, and this is regarded as the main cause of orthostatic hypotension in older people.

📄 Case history

Henry was an 80-year-old man who had had three falls in the preceding 2 months. On each occasion he had simply lost his balance and toppled over. There was no giddiness or loss of consciousness. He complained that over the preceding 2 years his legs had become progressively weaker, and that his balance had steadily deteriorated.

Twelve years earlier he had been found to have cancer of the left parotid gland (the gland on the side of the face that produces saliva). This had been removed surgically, and he had had a course of 30 radiotherapy treatments to this area.

He had wasting of the muscles of his legs, which were weak. Coordination in his legs was poor, and he did badly in tests of proprioception (position in space).

An MRI scan of his neck showed a normal spinal cord and brain. By the time he came back for review, he was more unsteady and had developed numbness in both feet. He now had mild orthostatic hypotension.

Nerve conduction studies confirmed that he had degeneration of his peripheral nerve fibres, called peripheral neuropathy. As so often happens, no cause was found for this.

He had a course of physiotherapy and education about falls, and was given a frame to make him steadier when walking. No specific treatment is available. Over the following year his condition stabilized. He was left with permanent unsteadiness on walking, but deterioration had stopped.

14

Osteoporosis and falls

> **→ Key points**
>
> The combination of falls and osteoporosis leads to fractures in later life.
>
> Osteoporosis is an abnormal thinning of the bone that leads to a susceptibility to fractures.
>
> Certain fractures are much more common with osteoporosis, when they are caused typically by low impact injuries:
>
> ◆ vertebral fracture (spine)
>
> ◆ fractured neck of femur (hip)
>
> ◆ wrist fractures
>
> ◆ pelvic fractures
>
> ◆ fractured neck of humerus (upper arm)
>
> ◆ fractured fibula (ankle)
>
> ◆ fractured fifth metatarsal (foot).
>
> Osteoporosis can be treated and its progression slowed.

Rugby players and footballers fall over all the time, sometimes after being knocked down with great force. They get up and run on, and only rarely are they injured by the fall. In older people the chances of a fall resulting in a broken bone are very greatly increased. There are certain types of fracture that are seen almost entirely in older people and which occur very rarely in the young.

Humpty Dumpty ended up in pieces not just because he had a great fall, but also because he had a very thin fragile shell. It is the combination of falls and abnormally thin bones which lead to such damage in elderly people. This process of thinning of the bones with age or with certain medical conditions is called osteoporosis.

What is osteoporosis?

Throughout life the body's bone structure is constantly renewed, with old bone being absorbed and new bone being laid down. Up to about the age of 40 more bone is put down than is absorbed. After that the process goes into reverse, and the bones start to become thinner (Figures 14.1 and 14.2). In women, this process accelerates after the menopause. Eventually enough bone has been lost for fractures to occur with minor injuries. Once this level of bone thinness is reached, it is described as osteoporosis. The diagnosis of osteoporosis depends upon measuring the density of bone using special equipment.

A statistically significant drop in the density of bone found in these measurements, compared with what would be expected in young adults (called the T score), is considered to be diagnostic of osteoporosis. Another score—the Z score—relates the bone density to that of other people of the same age, and is no longer used to determine treatment.

The diagnosis of osteoporosis can be made:

◆ on clinical grounds, in the presence of osteoporotic fracture

◆ by DEXA scanning to obtain a 'T score'.

There are a number of conditions which cause osteoporosis to develop more rapidly. The most common of these is the use of steroid tablets such as prednisolone. These are used to treat a number of illnesses such as asthma, arthritis, and polymyalgia rheumatica (also called giant cell arteritis or temporal arteritis). When treatment with steroids is prolonged, bone loss is inevitable. However, it can be diminished or even prevented by taking treatment for osteoporosis at the same time.

(a) (b)

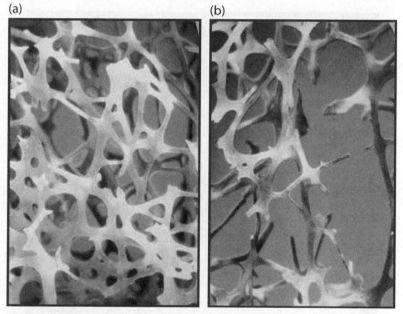

Figure 14.1 (a) Normal bone (age 20–50). (b) Osteoporotic bone (age 60+). Courtesy of Graham Russell.

Common fractures due to osteoporosis

The key feature of osteoporotic fractures is that they often result from surprisingly low-energy injuries. They are often collectively termed 'low-impact fractures'.

Vertebral fractures By far the most common type of fracture that results from thinning of the bones is crumbling of the vertebrae. This results in older people losing height, and older people becoming more and more bent forward when they stand up. The upper back develops a curve, which is called a dowager's hump or, in medical terms, a kyphosis. While many of these bones collapse painlessly and people develop this condition without becoming aware of it happening, in other cases the collapsed bone can be extremely painful. It is estimated that only one in three such fractures are ever diagnosed. Osteoporosis can give rise to chronic and intractable back pain (although, even in those with osteoporosis, back pain is commonly due to osteoarthritis of the back). Treatment of this process as soon as it is diagnosed can lead to it being slowed very considerably, although not completely.

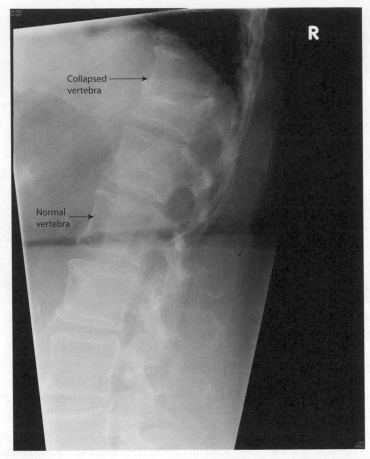

Figure 14.2 An X-ray of the back in side view showing collapse of a vertebral body. This can be seen at the top of the image where the vertebra appear smaller than the ones lying below.

📋 Case history

Hillary was an 85-year-old woman who was admitted following a fall at home, following which she was unable to stand and had pain in her left groin.

She was found to have severe orthostatic hypotension. She had been started on amitriptyline 50 mg at night as a sleeping tablet 5 years previously. The amitriptyline was stopped, and her blood pressure returned to normal.

In the period that she had been taking the amitriptyline she had fallen several times and had sustained two broken hips, a broken humerus, and a broken wrist. X-rays on the current admission showed that she had a fractured pelvis, and also had four vertebral fractures that she had acquired in the past, of which she was unaware.

She required 3 weeks in hospital to regain her mobility. In this time she managed to sleep reasonably well without the need for a sleeping tablet.

She was started on treatment for osteoporosis with calcium and vitamin D, and alendronate. The alendronate caused indigestion, and was changed to strontium ranelate. She made a good recovery, and when followed up 6 months later had not had any more falls.

Cases like this, where an unnecessary medication is causing multiple fractures, without the patient ever receiving treatment for osteoporosis, are far too common.

Fractured neck of femur (broken hip) is the most feared of the common fractures. It is three times more common in women than in men. It is usually the consequence of a fall onto the hip. Invariably an operation is required to repair or replace the hip joint. The outlook following this fracture is not good, with 20–25 per cent of victims dying within a year (frequently because they are reaching the end of their lives anyway, and have many other things wrong with them). About half of patients are not well enough afterwards to go back to living in their own homes, and many are left with chronic pain and serious disability.

Table 14.1 Lifetime risk of fracture for a 45-year-old white person

	Risk (%)	
	Female	Male
Shoulder	13	4
Forearm	21	5
Hip	23	11
Spine	15	9
Any of the above	47	24

Wrist fracture is usually the result of using an outstretched hand to break a fall. Typically both the bones of the forearm break just above the wrist, when the term 'Colles' fracture' is used.

Pelvic fractures are usually the consequence of a fall. The ring of bone at the front of the pelvis (the pubic ramus) snaps in two places, resulting in pain on weight bearing. There are usually no long-term consequences, and generally it heals completely. It usually results in a period of immobility until the pain of the fracture settles. This is normally between 2 and 4 weeks.

Fractured neck of humerus is a break of the upper arm just below the shoulder joint. It takes a long time to heal, and few people regain normal use of the shoulder joint. The arm is left to hang down in a sling, and heals over a few weeks.

Fractured fibula usually results from a slip or trip. The fibula is the smaller bone in the lower leg, on the outer side of the ankle joint. The fracture occurs just above the ankle joint. In most cases treatment involves having the leg in plaster or an orthopaedic boot for 12 weeks.

Osteoporotic fractures in women result in the use of more hospital bed days than diabetes, heart attacks, or breast cancer. To put the figures in Table 14.1 in perspective, the lifetime risk of breast cancer is about 11–13 per cent. Osteoporotic fracture is much more probable, but is not given nearly as much prominence in the media.

Those who have had one osteoporotic fracture are at increased risk of having another:

♦ after one fracture, the risk of another is increased fivefold

- after two fractures it is increased sevenfold

- after three fractures it is increased 27-fold.

Anyone who has had an osteoporotic fracture should be assessed for treatment before their life is blighted by the pain and disability caused by further fractures.

Treatment of osteoporosis

The prevention of osteoporosis should start in childhood by ensuring a healthy balanced diet, rich in calcium and vitamin D, with plenty of exercise and exposure to sunlight. This will ensure that the skeleton has the best chance of entering adulthood with the right amount of calcium, so that when it starts to lose bone, there is plenty there to start with.

Most adults do not have sufficient vitamin D, and this seems to be one of the main causes of osteoporosis in the older age group. Supplementation of vitamin D and maintaining a high calcium intake from middle age onwards will diminish the chances of osteoporosis developing in later life.

Once osteoporosis has been diagnosed, treatment is with supplements of calcium and vitamin D, together with specific treatments to strengthen the bone. The usual treatment is a type of drug called a bisphosphonate. This is taken once a week and is taken up by the bone, where it stays for months or years. Newer drugs have been developed that can be given by injection once a year.

Strontium ranelate is a milky drink that is taken daily, and is as effective as a bisphosphonate. It is easier to take, and does not cause the stomach upsets that some people have with bisphophonates.

Tetraperatide is a new development, which is too expensive for regular use at present. It consists of synthetic fragments of parathyroid hormone, which regulates bone metabolism. It can have a dramatic effect in improving the skeleton.

Each of these treatments reduces the chance of fractures due to osteoporosis. New treatments are being developed all the time, and this is a vibrant area of medical research.

Vertebroplasty

Where vertebral fractures cause persistent pain, injecting cement into the vertebra will stabilize the bone, thereby reducing pain. Stabilizing bone in this way is thought to diminish the chances of other vertebrae collapsing. Each time a vertebra becomes wedge-shaped, it increases the pressure on the front part of other vertebrae, making them more likely to collapse.

📄 Case history

Angela was an 82-year-old woman with Parkinson's disease who had sat down heavily on her bed while transferring from her chair. This immediately caused severe pain across the lower part of her back.

The pain persisted, and was unrelenting. It kept her awake at night, and prevented her walking. She had an MRI scan which showed osteoporotic collapse of her fourth lumbar vertebra. She was treated with painkillers which caused numerous side effects, including hallucinations, vomiting, and constipation. She was started on calcium and vitamin D, and alendronate 70 mg a week.

After 3 months she continued to be in severe pain. She had a vertebroplasty, with cement injected into the L4 vertebra. Her pain vanished overnight. She required a period of several months of rehabilitation to make up for the mobility she had lost while in pain, but eventually made a good recovery. She was delighted that she no longer required any painkillers.

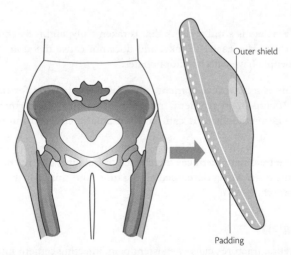

Outer shield

Padding

Figure 14.3 Hip protectors.

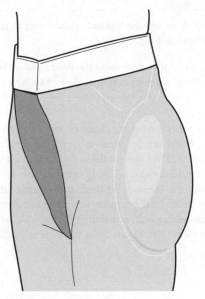

Figure 14.4 A garment containing hip protectors.

Hip protectors

Hip protectors consist of a pair of knickers containing a fibrous pad (like a footballer's shin pads) over each hip (Figures 14.3 and 14.4). When people are wearing them, a fall is unlikely to result in a hip fracture. The problem is that they are not particularly comfortable, and some types are difficult to get on and off to go to the toilet. Often they are not worn at night, which is a time of great risk of falls.

Hip protectors

♦ The early hopes for the use of hip protectors to prevent hip fracture has not been substantiated in subsequent large trials.

♦ A trial putting them on half of the residents of care homes in Northern Ireland showed no difference between those who had them and those who did not.

- A trial putting them on one hip only resulted in at least as many fractures in the protected hip.

- Apart from the fact that they raise the awareness of falls in the patient, family, and carers, they are not currently of proven benefit.

Only about a half of those who try them persist in the long term. Of those who do wear them, many do not wear them all the time and often fall when they are not being worn. They are useful in particular cases, for example when someone is falling frequently and is highly motivated to do whatever is possible to prevent a hip fracture. We suggest them to frequent fallers in care homes, where getting them on and off becomes the responsibility of the carers. Their greatest value in this setting is in reminding the carers that the patient is likely to fall and keeping them alert to ensuring the patient's safety.

15

Fear of falling

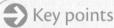 Key points

Fear of falling:

◆ causes an enormous amount of disability and dependency on others

◆ affects the family and carers

◆ is a common reason for going into a care home

◆ can be treated using exercise groups and cognitive behavioural therapy.

In order to stay upright we have to devote a certain amount of our attention to the processes of standing up or walking. Most of the time this takes place subconsciously, but at times, when our balance is threatened by a trip or a stumble, we suddenly become very conscious of what we have to do to stay upright. For a moment, we become afraid of falling.

Some people who feel unsteady when they stand become so scared of falling that the fear itself starts to have an effect on them. Many of these people have fallen before, and do not wish to repeat the experience. Roughly an equal number have not had any falls, but are nevertheless fearful of them.

Fear of falling causes a burden of disability as great as that caused by the injuries that result from falls.

Fear of falling, and of its consequences, need not be confined to the person at risk of falling. Frequently the family is afraid of them being left alone at home in case they should fall, and encourages them to give up their own home to go into a care home. Falling and fear of falling (without necessarily having had falls), when coupled with some degree of memory loss, are the main reasons that people go to live in care homes.

Questionnaires have shown that about a half of care home residents are fearful of falling, and about a quarter to half of the elderly population also admit to this fear. It is three times more common in women than men, and is more common in those with a history of depression or anxiety.

Several reasons are given for this quite rational fear. The most common is the loss of personal dignity involved—often it involves becoming dependent on someone else, possibly a complete stranger, to help you up. People are also fearful of falling and of being alone on the floor, unable to get up. Others fear the restriction of their activity that might be a consequence of injuries that they sustain.

> Fear of falling leads to a cycle of decline, limiting activities through fear. People then do less and less over a period of time as they become less fit, weaker, and less confident. This leads to greater unsteadiness and increased fear.

Overcoming the fear of falling

There are several approaches to overcoming the fear of falling, which should be used together.

- Improve strength and balance through exercise and balance training, which ought to make falls less likely.

- Ensure that the right walking aids have been considered, and that domestic hazards have been minimized.

- Teach people about falls, and explore their own fears and anxieties. This is often done within a group.

- Teach people how to get up again after a fall.

- Consider how they would summon help if they lay injured on the floor. Encourage the use of pendant alarms, which are reassuring to both the older person and the family.

A large part of the benefit of exercise classes is to boost people's confidence. Exercise has a small, but important, benefit in improving strength. Carrying out exercises and doing day-to-day tasks under supervision or in a group encourages people to do these things more freely at home once again. Usually they are things that they have done all their adult lives without thinking about them, but have stopped doing because of the anxiety they have about falling. Time and again we hear that after coming to our classes people have started going out to do their own shopping for the first time in years.

In the groups we try to educate people about why they fell, and teach them about their own individual risk factors. For many people, it is not understanding why they fell that makes them fearful. Educating people about their fears, explaining them, and getting them to understand them and look at them differently is known as 'cognitive behavioural therapy', and it has a good track record in several fields of medicine. Here it is used to address unrealistic concerns about falling, and to give insight into thoughts, feelings, and behaviours that result from fear, and which make the situation worse. Such an approach has a proven benefit, but is limited to those who are sufficiently mobile and sufficiently mentally able to benefit.

16

How do falls affect the family and carers?

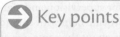 Key points

Who is affected?

- The spouse or partner

- Daughters, less commonly sons

- More distant relatives

- Friends

- Neighbours and other 'informal carers'

- Paid carers.

Falls can have a dramatic effect on the lives of those who fall. Their effect on family, friends, and carers is often as great. There are several aspects to this:

- fear and anxiety about future falls

- the need for supervision day and night

- the effects of falls that have already occurred

- the need for care to cope with loss of independence.

The faller may be scared of falling. Some fallers will limit their activity to diminish the risk of falls, and will do whatever is necessary to prevent them. Others are not concerned about the risk of further falls—it is their family and friends who are concerned about them.

Often the family would like their relative to be supervised so as to diminish falls, or to ensure that there is someone available to help when falls occur. Unless there is someone from the family available in the home who is free to do this, or someone can be hired to live in, a care home may be seen to be the answer. The patient often does not want to go into a care home, and continues at home unsupervised.

Following a fall, an injury may have led to some loss of the ability to do every-day things. Washing, dressing, shopping, cooking, and getting about freely may no longer be possible. Someone else has to step in to help, and an additional burden is put on them. The person who is likely to be most affected by falls is the husband, wife, or partner, if there is one. They usually live in the same house and do whatever is necessary to help. The need for supervision and vigilance may extend round the clock. They may have to provide help with care to an extent that stretches their limits. Often the spouse is about the same age as the patient, and may not be very well themselves.

How do falls affect the spouse? It depends upon many factors.

♦ The quality of their relationship.

♦ Is one (or both) of them confused or disabled? The spouse looking after the faller may be in need of care themselves.

♦ How fit each of them is—their level of independence in everyday tasks.

♦ Their psychological make-up. Is one of them an anxious person, or do they keep things in perspective?

♦ Their previous experience of falls and injuries.

♦ Their level of knowledge of what to do if a fall occurs and how pre-pared they are.

♦ The arrangements for summoning help should it be required.

The spouse will be affected by having to be constantly vigilant and constantly reminding the patient to take care. They will be anxious about the possibility of another fall, for which they may feel responsible. This responsibility lasts day and night, with no days off. This is a very stressful situation.

If there has already been an injury, then it will have had physical and mental consequences. It may have caused disability, and the patient may no longer be able to perform everyday tasks, either for a short period until an injury recovers or perhaps forever, as they may have lost the ability to do some things in a way that will not recover.

📄 Case history

William and Jane were both in their early nineties, and lived together in a large house. They had been completely independent, and William was still able to drive. Jane's walking was limited following a hip replacement that had not gone well 2 years previously.

One evening, William collapsed in the bathroom. Jane heard a loud crash, and went upstairs to find him lying on the floor groaning. She tried to get him up, but in doing so she fell herself and broke her left upper arm. Neither of them was able to get up, or to summon help, and they spent the night on the floor. Their cleaner found them when she called in the following morning.

William was very ill; he had had a small heart attack, and had a severe urinary infection leading to septicaemia. He slowly responded to treatment, but spent weeks recovering in hospital.

At the time of discharge 5 weeks later he was able to get up out of a chair with help, and to take a few steps with the help of a frame. His memory had deteriorated, and he was muddled at times (something that had probably started before he came into hospital, although it had not been noticed before his admission).

Jane had broken the head of her humerus at the shoulder, and had to keep her arm in a sling for several weeks. She was no longer able to wash or dress herself, and had difficulty managing the toilet independently. She was unable to use a walking frame because of her arm injury, and her walking had deteriorated. She was able to walk a few metres with a stick, but could no longer manage the stairs.

Their only daughter lived in another part of the country, and had a disabled husband to look after. The choice for William and Jane was either to go into a care home, or to employ someone to look after them at home.

A stair lift was installed, and an agency provided carers to live with them. The carers helped them with washing and dressing, and coming downstairs, and cooked for them.

This double fall changed this couple's life forever. It resulted in both of them losing their independence. Both required a long period in hospital.

As neither of them had fallen before, falls prevention would not have been something they would have contemplated prior to this event. They would probably not have accepted advice from an occupational therapist to make alterations to their home to make things safer, as both saw themselves as being fit and able. They would have been much better off if they had been able to summon help through an alarm system after falling, but each thought that the other would be there to help them if they fell ill.

ⓘ The wife's perspective

Henry is 84, and lives in a house with his wife who is fit and able, and a few years younger. He has orthostatic hypotension that has not responded to treatment, and has fallen regularly a few times a month for the last 4 years. He says his legs feel like lead, and he has great difficulty walking more than a few steps, which he does holding a frame tightly for support.

His wife says that she lives in terror of his falls. He is a big man, and when he falls he cannot get up, and she says that she is powerless to help him. Depending on the time of day, she calls the neighbours or her daughter, but during the working day or at night she has to call an ambulance so that the paramedics can get him up.

Mercifully, he has never suffered a serious injury despite countless falls. He makes no effort to protect himself as his feet crumple beneath him. A few times he has hit his head, and has had bumps and bruises. Above all, it is the inconvenience of his falls that worries her, and the fear that one day he will hurt himself.

When she goes out to the shops during the day he is left alone sitting in the chair. He is quite happy to stay and wait for her return, and makes no effort to move. Carers come in and help her get him in and out of bed, but she manages to look after him on her own for the rest of the time.

Children usually live separately from their parents, and have their own busy lives. There may be an expectation that they will provide supervision and care, but this is often impossible for them. Worries about their parents' safety and about their ability to look after themselves can cause an enormous amount of anxiety. They can only provide help to a significant extent if they live nearby. The further away they are, the more likely it is that someone else will have to be employed to provide help in the house, or that the patient will have to move house—either closer to the children, or to somewhere that provides a degree of supervision or care. This might be in a sheltered accommodation complex or a care home. The financial implications of providing this level of care are another source of stress and anxiety.

ⓘ The daughter's perspective

Jane is 95, and her daughter Jenny lives 2 hours drive from her. Jane has a mild dementia, a tendency to become dehydrated through not drinking, and has had several falls. Below is Jenny's account of the problems this creates.

There is no doubt that living away from your elderly loved one has mental and physical repercussions that come as a huge surprise. You discover that you have responsibility for your loved one without having control of them. And you discover that you have no training or preparation for the situation.

The temptation is to jump into the car every time you feel things are not quite right, or there is no reply from the phone. Not so disastrous when you are 2 hours away, but friends have a situation where their elderly mothers are on a different continent, and for them the fears are as real and even less manageable. In these cases well-meaning friends are often quick to alert the absent daughter that their mother is much worse/acting very strangely/has caused mayhem in the town/needs looking after.

Mentally you feel very alone when taking decisions especially on topics such as what level of care is needed, what is available, and what might be acceptable.

There are not really any friends of Mum's that can be relied on for practical help (they are dead or old and infirm themselves).

Interestingly, females without children seem to feel the agony and responsibility more acutely than men, or women who've had children.

In discussions with others, it is clear that we all feel guilt; we believe that, however much we do, we are not doing enough. I learned to live with this by doing a deal with myself. I worked out how much time I could afford to spend with Mum and still have a life. The deal was that if I delivered on that, I would not allow myself to feel guilty.

There is also a danger of family discord—why am I doing all the worrying, caring, travelling? Or resentment if another family member lives nearby and you, the distant sibling, tries to interfere. I have found that the only way to manage this is to realize that you have no choice but to do what you are comfortable with. After all, you will have to live with yourself and the decisions you have made.

One lives constantly in an anxiety bubble. Sometimes this is tolerable and other times it is deeply distressing.

I found that I dreaded the phone ringing when it was the time that the carer was due at Mum's. I dreaded phoning Mum and getting no reply—I feared that she had fallen, was ill, etc. In fact, normally she had fallen asleep and not heard the phone.

I dreaded phoning and getting a constantly engaged signal, fearing that she had fallen and knocked the phone off the hook. In fact, all too often she had been on the phone and not put it back properly.

Practically, you can't make personal plans with any certainty.

You don't look forward to anything in case something happens to Mum and you have to change plans/let others down.

You are reluctant to take on other commitments because Mum takes priority. My brother and I make sure we are never out of the country at the same time.

In my case I am hugely fortunate that I no longer have work commitments and so can afford to devote time to Mum. And now we have a wonderfully caring and capable carer/housekeeper living with Mum which has eased the pressure.

I am very lucky that I have friends who can sympathize and help by visiting Mum. Most importantly, I can appreciate that the overall effect has been very positive for me. The time spent with Mum has been an unexpected blessing, one of the highlights of my life. We've developed a new and very close relationship which would never have come about had she not become the fragile elderly relative.

ℹ The daughter's perspective

Sheena lives in Abingdon, and her elderly mother lived in Edinburgh. Here is her account of her mother's falls.

Early on a Friday morning, I received a call from Mum's neighbour, who informed me that my mum had fallen and had cut her head. An ambulance had been called and she was taken to A&E. The next hour was very long and your mind goes into overdrive, imagining all the nasty things which could happen. I had her dead and buried before I was able to contact A&E. Once I managed to get through to A&E, it was difficult to speak to someone who could tell me anything. Eventually I spoke to someone, who told me that her injuries were actually worse than I had first feared, and that she had broken her hip.

Then you think, do I go up, or do I wait? A very unsettling time. You can't focus on anything as your mind whirls round and round.

More information was forthcoming once she had been moved to the ward, and the pending operation clinched the decision to go up. The relatives in the USA also had to be informed, with endless calls back and forth. Once the decision had been made to go up, you are not totally settled, as you are unsure what to expect.

Once I saw Mum, some of my worries disappeared, as I felt she was in the best place. Then you start to worry about her long-term future. Mum fortunately made it home in time for her family in the USA coming over. A care package was also set up initially for her with help in the morning and evening.

About 3 weeks later, and about 5 days after I returned from my second visit, she fell again. Initially she was taken to the Rehab hospital, but because she appeared to be in terrible pain, once there she was transferred to A&E again. After another hip operation, I travelled back up to Edinburgh again. I think the worry was worse the second time round; another operation in a short space of time and if there were problems with managing at home before, what would it be like this time. She worked hard on her mobility but didn't quite make it. A home visit was not as good as hoped. Being a distance away too, you don't get told how the home visit really went. After a lot of pushing for answers, Mum made the decision that her next step was a care home. Initially I thought no, my Mum is too alert, but she had made the right choice.

Mum was happy to move down to this area. The hunt for a care home was the next problem. We looked round quite a number—good ones and some I would not consider.

We now have Mum settled in a care home, and it has made life a lot easier. She took a while to settle; everything is so different away from your own home. I know that she is being well looked after. The care home is excellent at contacting me if there is a medical problem and will contact her GP straight away. I still worry when I receive a call from the home, but knowing that I am only 20 minutes away does help.

Relatives and friends are often a part of the informal network of care that an older person develops. The care provided by friends and neighbours is usually at a lower level of intensity than what might be expected of spouses or children, such as help with the shopping, cleaning, or tasks that stop short of providing direct personal care. It is uncommon for friends to be able to provide 24-hour supervision or any direct care, and if a fall results in a loss of independence, it usually becomes necessary for formal paid help to be organized.

Faced with a relative who is falling at home, there is pressure to do something. The situation is an unfamiliar one, and it is difficult to know how to approach the problems it poses. Certain things are common to most people in this predicament, and in general such situations need:

◆ an assessment of risk

◆ an acknowledgement of that risk by those involved

◆ a consideration of the factors that influence the provision of care and supervision in the future.

Assessing the risks

To estimate the risks associated with falling we need to consider several things:

◆ the likelihood of having a fall

◆ the chance of an injury resulting from any fall

◆ the probable severity of that injury.

The likelihood of having a fall cannot be known for certain, but the more falls have already occurred, the more likely it is that they will continue with a similar frequency. Once everything possible has been done to prevent falls and to make the home safe, this risk will have been minimized, but may still be significant.

The chances of an injury occurring depend on where the falls happen. Stairs and areas with many sharp edges or hard floors (kitchens and bathrooms) pose particular risks. The risk of fracture depends on many things, among them the presence of osteoporosis, which makes bones weaker.

Managing the risks

◆ Assessing whether anything in the current situation is amenable to change.

◆ Making the risk explicit: a discussion with all concerned as to what the estimated risks are, and an exploration of the attitudes of the older person and the family to that level of risk.

◆ Acknowledging the risk and its consequences—considering how the risks affect everyone concerned. Does Mum realize what impact her risk of falling is having on her daughter's life?

Minimizing the risks

Have steps been taken to diagnose and manage the cause of the falls, assess the need for and encourage the use of walking aids, ensure a safe environment, and ensure effective ways of summoning help? Has everything been done to make things as safe as they can be?

Can risk be minimized with the patient in their current home? What can be done, and what would the patient accept in terms of care and supervision.

Once everything has been done to minimize the risks, discussions tend to be about help and supervision at home, or on moving to a different home. This may be somewhere nearer other members of the family who wish to and are able to provide support, or to a more supervised home—either sheltered accommodation or a care home.

What factors influence decisions about future care and supervision?

The benefits of not making changes

Disruption affects older people much more than the young, and moving house is a particular stress. A familiar environment is one in which the hazards are known, and successful strategies for dealing with them may have been developed. Moving to a new home poses particular risks of falling in the first few weeks.

The loss of social contacts on moving to a new area can have a deleterious effect, and some people move to another part of the country to be nearer their family, only to find themselves more socially isolated than they were before. Not all such moves are a success.

Moving often involves a change in the doctors, nurses, and carers involved. This can have a significant effect for better or worse. For those who feel they are well looked after by people they know and trust, the step into the arms of strangers is daunting.

Often it is easier simply to increase the amount of input to the home, but by the time such discussions arise, the situation has often become too precarious for staying at home to be a safe or acceptable option.

Many older people object strongly to having people come into their home to supervise them. They may lack insight as to what this supervision is for, and may object to paying for such services.

What burdens are being put on others?

Usually the burden of care and anxiety falls upon the family and carers. Most commonly caring is in addition to work and family commitments. It may have effects upon their own family and relationships. The burdens may be physical, psychological, or financial.

Autonomy

The patient has a right to make their own decisions, even if these might appear irrational or unsafe in the eyes of others. Persuasion can be tried, but the patient's decision has to be respected.

Only when someone is incapable of understanding what their situation really is can others start to make decisions on the basis of the patient's best interests. This would almost always involve input from medical specialists.

A frequent problem is that the patient sees their risk differently—and usually more optimistically—than others do. Sometimes poor memory or confusion mean that the risk cannot be properly understood or assessed by the patient, who wants nothing to change in the face of risks that are considered unacceptable by everyone else.

17

How to improve strength and balance

→ **Key points**

Exercise will increase strength and stamina predictably, but its effect on balance is less certain.

Balance training involves:

- developing the appropriate use of corrective movements at the ankle and the hips, and the use of effective steps to restore stability

- improving posture

- diagnosing and improving abnormal gait

- re-training the brain to make the best use of sensory inputs

- improving strength and stamina

- improving confidence

- making appropriate use of walking aids.

Anything that we do to improve our levels of fitness and stamina, and to improve the strength of our legs, is likely to make us more stable. In general, the benefit from exercise classes is partly through improving strength, but to a large extent is through boosting confidence. A great deal of the disability in fallers, and even in those elderly people who have not fallen, is caused by a lack of confidence.

Exercise needs to be regular to be of continuing benefit through improving strength and stamina. Getting benefit out of exercise involves learning which exercises to do, and then having the determination to do them regularly. Studies looking at the benefit of exercise classes show that they need to be continues for at least 9 months to really make a difference.

> A vital role of exercise classes is to improve confidence.

There is a considerable body of research showing the benefits of exercise in people who fall. Some of these exercises are concerned with improving muscle strength and stamina, while others are for improving balance or flexibility. Some, such as t'ai chi, the Chinese balance exercises, have caught the public imagination.

While there is good evidence that exercises to improve strength are successful in doing so, poor balance is often due to underlying illness or disability, and in many cases the response to training is disappointing.

> Balance is to some extent task specific. Someone who is good at riding a bicycle will not automatically be able to walk a tightrope.
>
> Tests that measure one aspect of balance correlate poorly with the results of other balance tests in the same patient. Balance training also needs to focus on specific tasks.

The control of balance

Balance control is complex and can be deranged in many ways. It involves being able to decide upon and to perform movements that keep our centre of gravity within an area that is vertically above our feet.

The movements that keep us upright are both conscious and unconscious. They may be made to anticipate a change in position, or in response to some outside force that has changed our balance, such as being pushed. Whereas the first movements are planned, the second are automatic.

Standing upright is the easiest posture to maintain—it uses up the least energy. When we stand, we do not stay completely still, but sway slightly from side to side. The amount that we can sway before we become unstable diminishes with age. To remain upright, and to make minor adjustments to our position so as to keep our centre of gravity above our base of support, we use three different types of movement:

◆ moving at the ankles

◆ moving at the hips

◆ taking a step.

> The area over which we are stable is termed the **base of support**. When standing, it corresponds roughly to an area that can be drawn around where our feet are placed on the floor. When sitting, the base of support is very much larger, both backwards and forwards and side to side.

Ankle movements

The ankle is used for small movements to respond to a minor disturbance of balance. Most of the body's natural sway occurs at the ankles. For the body to rebalance by moving backwards or forwards at the ankle joint requires an adequate range of movement in the joint and good strength in the muscles around it. For this to work, a firm surface below the feet is required, or else the feet will dig into the surface, rather than the body moving its position. An adequate level of sensation in the feet and ankles is also necessary so that the body knows how much movement there should be, and how much has taken place once a movement has been started.

Patients with arthritic ankles, muscle weakness in the legs, or sensory loss due to nerve damage from whatever cause will have an impairment of ankle movements. Older women in particular lose flexibility in their ankles with age. This is less marked in men, which may reflect a woman's lifetime of wearing fashionable footwear.

Hip movements

Movements at the hip can be both backwards and forwards, and side to side in order to restore the position of the centre of gravity above the feet. They are used when larger movements of the centre of gravity have taken place.

Once again, they are dependent on a good range of movement at the hip joint, and good muscle strength around the joint. This is often lost once the hip becomes arthritic. The buttock muscles are important in maintaining sideways stability and preventing unwanted sideways movement at the hip. Anything that affects their strength will also affect stability at the hip, and may lead to falls.

> A loss of flexibility in the back and neck, and also at the shoulder, are associated with an increased risk of falls. In particular, the loss of movement at the ankle joint with age impairs the ability to maintain balance by ankle movement.

Taking a step

Minor adjustments of position can be made at the ankles or the hip, but when a significant change in position needs to be made, we have to take a step. This happens whenever the centre of gravity is moved outside the base of support, and the step results in a new base of support. This occurs when the centre of gravity has moved too far, or when the change in position is very rapid.

Retaining balance by taking a step is dependent on the ability to move the legs quickly, and anything that affects muscle strength or slows reaction times will affect the speed of this response. Anything that affects lower limb strength, or mental or physical reaction times, will affect both how quickly you can take a step and how well judged the step is. When taking steps to compensate, it is much more common for older people to hit one leg with the other, causing them to trip over their own feet.

As people grow older, their assessment of what step needs to be taken is less accurate, and they tend to take a number of smaller stuttering steps where a younger person would take a single confident step. Commonly one of the steps that is made is backwards or forwards, and another to the side, to widen the base of support. Older people resort to taking a step, rather than a hip or ankle movement, earlier than do the young. It takes a smaller challenge to result in a step, and the steps are then less effective at restoring balance; they are less well judged and multiple.

Factors which may contribute to these smaller poorly controlled steps include the following.

◆ The buttock muscles, which control sideways movement, may be weak and have to work at the limit of their capability.

◆ Many older people have impaired sensation from their feet, or even a neuropathy causing a significant loss of nerves to the feet. Experiments in younger people show that numbing the feet results in multiple steps, and this sensory loss in older people may contribute to their step pattern.

In real life these strategies are used in whatever combination is necessary, rather than one being selected over another. Exercises aim to practise coordinating strategies and getting responses of the right size.

Once these movements to restore balance start, sensations from the body, the eyes, and the inner ear tell us how effective the movements have been, and allow us to decide what further movements might be necessary. The brain has to plan these actions so that the right groups of muscles can be activated in the right order and with the appropriate force.

Sensory inputs are vital in telling us whether the movement we have made has been successful in restoring balance, and helping us plan the next step. Vision plays a key role once we are walking in assessing whether we are well balanced, anticipating changes that we can see ahead of us, and avoiding obstacles. The brain needs to organize the right groups of muscles to work at the same time to achieve these movements.

Dividing attention between two tasks leads to one of them being performed less well. Car drivers are not allowed to use a mobile phone because speaking into it distracts their concentration, not because they have to use one hand to hold the phone. This phenomenon becomes more noticeable with increasing age, and a larger proportion of the brain's resources is needed to maintain balance. Any distraction—speaking, carrying something, looking around—is likely to increase the chances of a fall.

> Many older people are instinctively aware of the way that distractions threaten balance. They stop and stand still whenever they have to talk.

Gait and balance training
Controlling the centre of gravity

Abnormal posture is very common, and often the sense of what is vertical is lost, leading to an abnormal (and unbalanced) standing posture, with the head bent down, round shoulders, the pelvis tilted back, and the knees slightly bent. Many people lean slightly to one side, or put more weight on one side of the body. This is very common in those with arthritic joints, those who have had a stroke, and those who have had surgery or an injury to a limb.

Exercises to restore control over the centre of gravity aim to maintain a better upright position when sitting or standing. They help to feel how the centre of gravity should be controlled when still and when moving, both consciously and subconsciously. They aim to help manage unexpected challenges to balance, and to handle two tasks at the same time.

Sensory inputs to balance

Vision, body sensation, and the vestibular system of the inner ear are the three sensory inputs that tell us about where we are in space. All these systems work less well with increasing age, and in addition each of them can be affected by common illnesses. Trying to show that training these systems will improve overall balance is difficult, but we do know that those who dance regularly have better balance than the rest of us. Regular use improves the function of most of the body's systems. What is certain is that, done properly, such exercises will contribute to increasing confidence, which is the main benefit of this training.

Movements to maintain posture

Training involves increasing awareness of the movements needed to rebalance position—at the ankle, at the hip, and taking a step. Training practises making the right movement, and encourages a movement of the right magnitude needed to restore balance.

Improving walking

Walking involves a complex series of actions as weight is transferred from one leg to another, and the body is moved forward. With age, the pattern of walking changes, and more time is spent in a stable position, with weight divided between both feet. The length of each step reduces, and the time taken to make the step increases.

There are three key components of walking: placing the foot on the ground and transferring weight onto it, standing on one leg once the other is raised, and bringing the trailing leg through to the front.

Putting the body's weight onto the forward foot is the most difficult part, because of the way the leg needs to absorb the shock of the foot hitting the ground. Vision is used to assess the surface on which the foot will be placed: Is it level? Is it slippery? Is it higher or lower? Sensation from the foot tells us when contact has been made, and whether the new surface feels safe and secure. Finally, weight is transferred onto the foot, using the leg and buttock muscles, and applying stresses to the joints.

The weight is then on one leg while the other is moved. This requires the leg muscles to be strong enough to take the whole weight on that leg. Joint pains can make muscles give way suddenly. A stumble can result in the need for a sudden increase in the amount of work the muscles have to do, exceeding their abilities. While on one leg, the body's weight is shifting and balance has to be readjusted. This position is unstable, and stability is only restored once the other leg hits the ground, offering more support.

Trips

Bringing the back leg through depends upon being able to move at the hips, knees, and ankles. The knee has to bend to raise the foot so that it clears the ground by about 1 cm. The foot has to be kept up so that the toe does not catch on the ground.

If swinging the other leg through results in the foot touching the ground, it causes a momentary delay in the planned movement, resulting in a loss of balance. This sort of trip is a common cause of falling, whether because of an uneven surface or something wrong with the leg.

The tendency for the foot to catch is more pronounced in people who have had a stroke. It is common for the affected leg to drag, or perhaps have a foot drop, where the muscles keeping the front of the foot up are affected; the toes may drag on the ground as the foot is moved. People who have had a hip replacement or a hip fracture often find that one leg is shorter than the other. When they are standing on the shorter leg, an extra effort has to be made for the long leg to clear the ground as it is brought forward.

When older people walk they tend to take steps that are of uneven length. When such irregular steps are combined with a tendency not to pick up their feet properly, it increases the chances of the foot catching on the ground, causing a stumble.

Vision

Vision is important during walking for several reasons. Together with the vestibular system, it allows us to keep our head in the right position. It lets us see what the surface is like ahead of us, and adjust our step accordingly. It allows us to see and then to avoid obstacles.

Improving strength and stamina

Muscle strength deteriorates gradually with age. People may live within their limitations, and have no great desire to become fitter until something happens that threatens their independence. They may then realize that exercise really is necessary to make them strong enough and confident enough to carry on at home, and to carry out the activities they have always done. Age is not a barrier to gaining strength through exercise. Older people are often very unfit to start with, and gain a great deal through doing just a small amount of exercise.

Ideally, such exercise should be built into everyday life and not be a separate event. This may involve making use of the upstairs toilet instead of one down-stairs, ensuring the benefit of several trips up the stairs a day (in those for whom it is safe to do so!), or walking to the corner shop for small items rather than driving to a supermarket.

Improving joint and muscle movement

The flexibility of muscles and joints deteriorates with age. This process involves thickening of the tissues that surround joints, and changes such as arthritis in the joint and weakness of the muscles around them. This leads to a diminished range of movement of most joints.

The mobility and stability of joints can be improved by strengthening the muscles that work around them. Daily exercises which put the major joints through their full range of movement will help to keep them flexible.

18

What is the role of falls groups and exercise classes?

→ Key points

Falls groups and exercise classes should follow a full medical assessment, as there may be a medical cause for the falls. Often the diagnosis and treatment of a medical problem, or a change in medication, is all that is needed to prevent further falls. Even in such cases, falls groups may be helpful in restoring confidence.

Balance exercises are concerned with:

- regaining control of the centre of gravity

- training the senses by reducing the input from other senses, forcing the use of the one that is being trained

- training the ankle, the hip, and step strategies

- changing the walking pattern

- improving strength and stamina

- improving confidence.

Falling affects people in different ways. There are many different potential causes of falls, and for most people there are several contributory factors. Falls groups are one way of handling this large number of people, who each have different problems. However, although their problems will not be the same, there are likely to be common themes.

Falls groups

Falls groups:

◆ are usually led by a therapist or a specialist nurse

◆ give time for the underlying causes of falls to be explained and explored

◆ a plan for treatment, which will be different for each individual, can be developed and implemented.

Everyone in the group was once able to walk safely; they are not being taught to walk again, but to do something they have done all their lives more safely and with greater confidence. The benefits of these classes are mostly in the confidence that it gives people to do things once again.

Treating people who have fallen involves getting to the bottom of what the cause, or causes, were for them. These will be different in each case. It follows that falls groups should follow a medical assessment that has explored the possible medical causes of falling.

Every faller will have their own pattern of problems that could have led to the fall, their own mental attitude to falling (which may depend on whether they injured themselves), and their own level of physical and mental function. Everyone will need a personalized approach to educating them about falls, training them about how to prevent further falls, and teaching them what to do if further falls do occur.

However:

◆ Not everyone will benefit from group work.

◆ Group work implies the ability to learn and to take an active part, and those with severe memory problems are unlikely to be helped (although they may still gain benefit from exercise classes).

◆ Those in whom a simple remediable cause for their fall has been found are unlikely to fall again, and may have no need of such treatment.

What happens in a falls group depends upon the patient's problems, and their physical state. Locally we run several different types of groups.

Falls groups are offered following a specialist assessment. There are several different types of falls groups.

◆ Balance and safety classes are offered to those at risk of further falls, and those who have lost confidence.

◆ Frail or housebound people are offered chair-based exercises, either in groups or in their own homes.

◆ Those at high risk of further falls are offered individual treatment in the day hospital.

◆ Fit and mobile people at low risk of falling attend exercise classes, with a course of discussions about falls.

Balance and safety classes

Those who have fallen and are at risk of further falls, or who have lost confidence attend our balance and safety classes following an assessment by our falls specialist.

◆ They are assessed by a physiotherapist to develop a personalized exercise programme.

◆ They have advice about walking aids and footwear.

◆ An occupational therapist assesses their ability to function at home, and arranges appropriate aids and adaptations in the house.

◆ Help with personal care is arranged if required.

◆ They have group discussions and education sessions. An instructor leads discussions about:

  ◆ the causes of falls

  ◆ how to prevent them

  ◆ how to maintain an active and healthy lifestyle

  ◆ appropriate footwear

  ◆ a balanced diet

  ◆ osteoporosis

  ◆ what assistance is available to them locally

  ◆ a wide variety of other issues, often those raised by members of the group.

There is good evidence that this group approach helps people to learn about falls and overcome their fears. It improves their confidence and their level of function. They start to go out more and to do more for themselves. It is one part of a successful strategy for reducing falls and fractures, but its contribution is hard to determine. It works, the patients like it, and the benefit is greater than the sum of its individual parts.

📄 Case history

Barbara was an 84-year-old woman with a long history of faints, occurring two or three times a year for over 40 years. In the last 5 years she had fallen about six times unrelated to fainting episodes.

She came to our balance and safety course for 8 weeks. She said: 'It made me more careful, and more aware of things that might make me fall. After a talk on dangers in the house I removed one of my rugs, and made sure the alarm cords all reached down to the floor. I do the exercises regularly. Some I do sitting in a chair, and others standing up holding on to the back of a chair. The course was definitely useful. It gave me more confidence. I can now walk for 20 minutes down to the shops, which I haven't been able to do for the last four years.'

Chair-based exercise classes

Those who are frail and housebound are unlikely to cope with the usual exercise classes, and are invited to sessions of chair-based exercises (Figures 18.1 and 18.2). The aim is:

◆ to improve the general level of stamina

◆ to strengthen the arms

◆ to provide psychological benefit from socializing and sharing their problems with others, as many older people lead very isolated lives

◆ to give an opportunity for their support networks of carers and social inputs to be explored and strengthened

◆ to provide education about what to do when they do fall

◆ to increase their confidence levels and, by overcoming irrational fears, improve their general level of function

◆ to check that they have appropriate walking aids and alarm systems

◆ to provide training in how to get up off the floor in case of a fall, and what to do if they cannot get up.

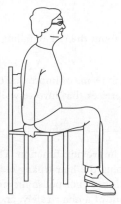

Chair march

- Sit tall
- Hold the sides of the chair
- Alternately lift your feet and place them down with control
- Build to a rhythm that is comfortable for you
- Continue for 30 seconds

Figure 18.1 Chair-based marching exercises. Illustration by Marion Lefebvre from *Strength and Balance Exercises for Healthy Ageing*, published by Help the Aged in 2006.

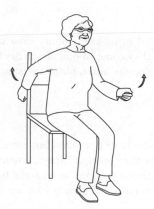

Arm swings

- Sit tall away from the chair back
- Place your feet flat on the floor below your knees
- Bend your elbows and swing your arms from the shoulder
- Build to a rhythm that is comfortable for you
- Continue for 30 seconds

Figure 18.2 Chair-based arm exercises. Illustration by Marion Lefebvre from *Strength and Balance Exercises for Healthy Ageing*, published by Help the Aged in 2006.

Chair-based exercise classes are helpful for those:

- who are very unsteady

- who would be put at risk of falling during exercise

- who are frail

- who are housebound (and are anxious about the risk of falling during unsupervised exercise).

While this is of some use, the main benefit in terms of improving balance and muscle strength must be found in exercises that involve walking or balancing.

Exercises that are done seated are aimed at improving function. They try to improve everyday movements, such as combing the hair (many older people have difficulty in raising their arms above their head) or polishing movements. There are exercises to teach people to get out of a chair safely, and to manage postural giddiness. The psychological benefits of this type of exercise are important, with many people being housebound and isolated. Frequently such exercise classes are the only time such people leave their homes.

Day hospital assessments

People who are at high risk of falling need to be seen sooner than we can provide a place in one of our groups, and they come to one of our day hospitals, where they are seen urgently by the falls specialists, physiotherapists, and occupational therapists.

Exercise classes

People who are at low risk of falling, or who have not fallen but are anxious about falling or wish to sustain or improve their level of fitness, attend exercise classes. These are followed by educational sessions as with the balance and safety classes. Exercise classes are primarily for people who are fit and mobile.

Regular exercise classes can be of use even to people with dementia, for whom few of the usual interventions to prevent falls can be applied.

To have continued benefit, the exercises need to be regular, and many day centres now offer exercise classes as part of their regular routine.

> Many older people come to us after a stay in hospital, often related to an injury they sustained when falling. Many have become 'deconditioned'— generally weak through lack of muscle use. It can take months for people to regain their strength following a period in bed in hospital. A week of bed rest results in the loss of 20 per cent of a person's muscle strength.

What do balance exercises involve?

Controlling the centre of gravity

These are exercises to re-train posture control. A variety of things can cause people to fail to stand up straight, or to tilt to one side, or to lose a sense of where their centre of gravity is. They are likely to have their centre of gravity towards one edge of their base of support when standing still, and will need only a small movement to make them unstable and more likely to fall.

The exercises involve moving the centre of gravity backwards and forwards and from side to side. Balance can be challenged by moving the body and the arms around, and a series of movements can be made which encourage an awareness of where the centre of gravity is and what needs to be done to restore it. Exercises can be made gradually more difficult in a variety of ways. They can start off seated, and then be repeated while standing, and then moving.

Seated exercises can be graduated:

- initially on a firm chair with a back support

- moving on to a stool without a back

- then to a soft surface, such as an exercise ball on a support to keep it still

- then the ball without support.

The exercises can be done:

- with the eyes open

- then in dim light or in dark glasses

◆ then with eyes shut

◆ the patient's attention can be divided by asking them to count or to speak during the exercise.

The patient can start with their arms on the chair or ball, progress to having their hands on their lap, and then keeping the arms across the chest, with each stage being more difficult than the last.

Training the senses

Exercises to train each of the senses are performed by trying to reduce the input of the others, forcing you to make more use of the one that is being trained.

Vision

Exercises to improve the way you use vision are done by decreasing the amount of sensation you have from your body. This can be done by sitting on a soft surface, such as an exercise ball, with the feet on a foam mat, or by standing on such a mat. An unstable surface, such as a rocker board, can also be used. The wobbly surface does not allow the brain to receive all the information it needs to assess position, and the emphasis falls on the eyes and the vestibular system. Alternatively, exercises can be done with a limited base of support, i.e. with the feet close together, or with one in front of the other, or even standing on one leg.

The exercises involve fixing the eyes on a distant point, and then introducing movements that would threaten balance—stretching or walking, and then progressing to carrying things, or to walking on tip-toes. The depth of the soft surface can be altered, or walking can be changed from marching on the spot to walking with varying step lengths.

Proprioception

Body sensation becomes increasingly important when vision is impaired, or when it is dark. Some people can walk reasonably well in the daytime, but are unsteady walking in the dark—their body sensation can be so impaired that they depend upon vision to maintain balance. This is usually seen in those with damage to their peripheral nerves.

Exercises involve sitting or standing on a firm surface, focusing attention on those parts of the body in contact with the floor or the chair. With eyes closed, balance has to be maintained while moving the arms, shifting weight, or reaching for things. Instead of closing the eyes, visual distraction can be used, trying to keep a steady position while following a moving object with the eyes.

Vestibular system

Training the use of the vestibular system involves doing exercises with the eyes shut, and on a soft surface to minimize the amount of body sensation. They start with trying to remain seated upright while sitting on an exercise ball, with the feet on a soft surface and the eyes shut.

The next step is to perform movements of the arms and legs while in this position. This can be done standing on a foam surface with the eyes shut, and then while walking on a foam surface with the eyes shut. Instead of closing the eyes, exercises can be done with visual distraction—looking at something, or performing some other visual task while trying to balance.

Ankle, hip, and step balance strategies

Most of the sway that takes place when you stand takes place at the ankles. By standing still, and swaying increasing distances from the upright position, the awareness of this movement can be increased.

The exercises can be made more difficult by repeating them while standing on a soft surface, and then by testing the response to a gentle push or pull. Closing the eyes adds to the difficulty of the task.

A moderate amount of movement away from the upright, or a more rapid movement, will result in balance being restored using the hips. Swaying backwards and forwards will use the ankle joints, but as movements are made more rapidly, and further backwards and forwards, the hips will come into play. Exercises can be made more difficult with an uneven surface.

Leaning forward as far as possible, and then a little further, results in a step being taken to change the base of support. Making these movements consciously and trying to adjust the length of the step helps to get used to making these movements. This can be repeated leaning backwards and to the sides.

The next level of exercises involves provoking situations in which balance is challenged by an outside force such as a push or a pull. This results in automatic responses, rather than the planned ones above. It is these responses that are the most useful in preventing a stumble becoming a fall. It is hoped that practising these movements in a controlled way during exercise sessions will result in their being used at the right moment at other times.

Exercises to improve walking

The aim of these exercises is to train people to adopt a pattern of walking that is flexible, and which can be changed to adapt to circumstances. It involves starting and stopping suddenly, walking with sudden changes in pace and in direction, and learning to cope with crowded spaces and obstacles. The exercises can be made more difficult by asking the patient to carry things, or by distraction through counting or talking.

Challenging the walking pattern in this way trains the ability to cope with real life situations, in which unexpected changes in what is going on around the patient cause moments of imbalance. The greatest benefit comes, once again, in increasing confidence in doing things, rather than teaching the ability to do new tasks.

Improving strength and stamina

In terms of walking and balance, it is the muscles of the leg that matter most. Exercises are aimed at strengthening the muscles of the buttocks, the thighs, the hamstrings, and those that move the foot up and down.

Exercises can start off in a sitting position, simply raising the leg at the hip, and then progress to standing up out of the chair. Standing exercises can be done using a support, such as squatting while holding on to a rail, or standing on toes and then on heels. As strength and confidence improve, so more complex exercises with increasing amounts of effort required can be done.

Improving movement around joints

Exercises aim to increase the range of movement by stretching the surrounding tissues. They need to be developed gradually and performed regularly. Exercises that involve sudden movements should be avoided. Movement at the neck and back, the shoulders, and the hips, knees, and ankles can all be improved by stretching exercises.

19

How can your world be made safer?

➔ **Key points**

◆ Causes of falls are divided into intrinsic and extrinsic factors.

◆ Alarm systems are vital for those who fall. Even those who can usually get themselves up may need help if they are injured by the fall.

◆ Certain actions are typically associated with falls—getting up at night, using the bathroom and kitchen, crossing the road, and anything that involves turning round present a significant risk.

◆ To prevent falls in the home requires an awareness of falls risk, and a willingness to change behaviour to do things more safely. Many things can be done differently in and around the house to increase safety.

◆ An occupational therapist can assess falls hazards at home, and recommend changes in behaviour and equipment that will diminish the risk of falls.

What is needed to maintain safety at home will be different for every individual, but there are things that older people tend to have in common, and changes that can be made which are of general benefit.

Above all, maintaining safety requires an awareness of the risk of falling, and a change in behaviour to minimize this risk consciously. Changes in behaviour are difficult for many people, as it is easy to forget about the risk of falling, particularly for those who have had only a few falls or whose memory is failing.

New routines have to be devised for tasks that used to be done without having to think about them. Plans have to be made to deal safely with a variety of situations. It is important to recognize which activities present a particular risk of falling.

Intrinsic and extrinsic factors causing falls

When looking at what might cause falls at home, possible contributory factors are divided into two groups—'intrinsic' and 'extrinsic'.

◆ Extrinsic factors mean those other than the person, namely things around them, chief of which is the home they live in.

◆ Intrinsic factors are those relating to the person. These might be poor vision, medication, confusion, or any one of the many factors detailed in this book.

One of the most common situations in which people fall is when getting up to go to the toilet at night. They have often been asleep, and are only half awake when they get up. It may be dark. They get out of a warm bed quickly, possibly provoking a significant drop in blood pressure on standing. They may have taken sleeping tablets, the effects of which will not yet have worn off. They then set off to the toilet forgetting to put on their glasses, without turning on the lights, and without their walking aids or slippers. The risk of falling at such a moment is enormous.

Trying to remember to modify your behaviour in the middle of the night is difficult, but several things can be planned beforehand. Having a decent pair of slippers available, having your stick or frame by the bed and your glasses placed conveniently nearby, and leaving a light on somewhere will all diminish the risk of falling. A commode by the side of the bed may be a good solution for those who fall repeatedly in such circumstances.

Turning round poses the greatest threat to balance, and is the movement most commonly associated with falls.

Most falls in the home occur in the bathroom, toilet, or kitchen—areas in which activities involve turning round. In addition, they are performed standing up and involve moving around in a confined space.

The other moments of particular risk are on getting out of a chair after prolonged sitting, and turning round quickly. Any change in position needs to be done slowly, while holding on to stable supports. Counting to 10 after standing up and before moving off will allow the brain to accustom itself to where it is in space, and for any changes in the blood pressure to settle, before balance is further challenged by trying to walk.

Changing position—and getting up and turning around—are hazardous because of the sudden change in the information reaching the brain. The eyes, the inner ear, and proprioception all take a few moments to give the brain sufficient information about its new position. At the same time the blood supply to the brain may have dropped with a drop in blood pressure, further impairing the brain's ability to assess where it is in space.

Making plans

Many everyday tasks around the house are potentially hazardous, and thinking about things beforehand can diminish the risk of falling.

Anything that involves climbing on to things, such as a stool or a chair, or reaching up to something represents a risk. Where possible, other people should be asked to perform these risky tasks. Changing light bulbs, taking curtains down for cleaning, even reaching up to hang out the washing are hazardous activities that are typically associated with falling.

Armchairs are often difficult to get out of because they are too low. They can be raised by putting blocks under each chair leg. There is a technique for getting out of a chair safely—slide your bottom forward, both arms on the arms of the chair, lean forward so that the weight is over the toes, and then push up with the arms to stand.

Fear of further falls is a constant factor for some people, while others face the real risk of falling without being concerned by it. Both groups might benefit from the use of alarm systems which they can activate to call for help if they do fall.

Inside the house

Many things can be done to make life at home safer:

In the kitchen

◆ Everyday items in the kitchen should be placed on convenient shelves that are easy to reach.

◆ A perching stool allows food to be prepared while sitting down, which may be safer.

Around the house

◆ Washing can be hung out on an airer rather than a clothesline.

◆ Getting up rapidly to answer the telephone is risky:

　◆ actions to reduce the number of unnecessary telephone calls diminish this risk

　◆ a mobile handset that you can keep by you at all times prevents the need to get up to answer the phone.

◆ Many homes are full of clutter on the floor, and simply removing this may have a great effect on improving safety and confidence.

In the bathroom

◆ Bathroom aids can be obtained to make getting in and out of the bath safer.

◆ Grab rails can be provided around the bath to assist with balance.

◆ Installing a shower stool or shower seat and rails to hold on to removes the need to stand in the shower.

◆ A strip wash by the basin may be easier than taking a shower.

In the toilet

◆ A raised toilet seat makes it easier to get up, as most toilet seats are a little too low.

◆ A frame around the sides of the toilet provides support while getting up and while adjusting clothing.

On the stairs

◆ Rails fixed to the walls for support may make it safer and easier to go up and down stairs.

◆ A rail around the newel post at the bottom gives an additional point to hold on to.

◆ Having a light on continuously above the landing at night makes it less likely that you will fall down the stairs.

◆ Once the stairs are no longer manageable, a stair lift can be fixed to the wall or the stairs, and is simple to use.

Outside the house

As people start to have recurrent falls, they go outside less and less frequently. However, many patients experience falls outside, and there are certain typical situations in which they occur. The most common reason given for a fall is an uneven pavement. Pavements in which there are many changes in levels, with drives and exits, or which are poorly maintained are a particular risk. The uneven surfaces put down at crossing places to help the visually impaired are a hazard for those with poor mobility.

Many patients fall at the kerbside. They fall either as they are stepping up onto the kerb, misjudging its height, or when they are setting off to cross the road. Looking one way and then the other to see if the road is clear is exactly the action that will challenge their balance most severely.

Travelling outside the home is always potentially hazardous. The sudden movement as a bus moves off causes people to lose balance and fall if they are not sitting down. This happens frequently, and bus companies are often sued by people injured in this way. For those who use taxis, it is often useful to build a relationship with a particular taxi company, which can get to know you and understand your problems and limitations.

> Bus drivers receive special training to make them aware of the hazards to older people of moving off too quickly. The bus driver should be aware of this risk, and reminding him to wait until you are sitting before moving off is a useful precaution.

In the winter, it is worth limiting trips outside to a minimum when the weather is bad. The same applies to particularly hot days in the summer. It is worth trying to get home earlier in the winter to avoid being out in the dark, and staying at home when the weather is bad. A gardening service may be helpful for clearing the front path in the summer, and keeping it free of slippery leaves in the autumn.

When walking outside, carrying a stick may provide a signal for others to warn them of your difficulties with walking or balance.

Walking on cycle lanes is hazardous, as cyclists approach quietly, and being startled by them as they pass may be enough to cause a fall. The same may happen with traffic noise, when turning too quickly can cause imbalance.

While risks at home cannot be completely removed, experience shows that heightening the patient's awareness of their risk has a major effect on reducing the number of falls that they have.

Sadly, those whose memory is impaired, and who cannot remember to do things differently, do not gain these benefits, unless they have someone there to remind them constantly.

The occupational therapist

A variety of risks can arise in the home, which can be removed or diminished. Usually this happens after an assessment by an occupational therapist, who might suggest a variety of aids and adaptations to the house. Typically, only about half of the recommendations made by therapists are ever acted upon by the patient. Not all older people like having a woman young enough to be their granddaughter coming to the house to tell them how to live their lives.

The occupational therapist's visit to the house has a further aim. It is to assess how safely various tasks are being done, and to suggest ways of doing things in a more secure manner. By reinforcing the need to focus on safety, therapists can diminish the chances of a fall.

As people grow older, they may need some physical help with tasks that they have done safely and confidently all their lives. It may be that the therapist recommends the help of someone coming to the house to assist with basic tasks such as getting up in the morning, washing, dressing, and the preparation of food.

Footwear

Footwear is implicated in many falls, but it is rarely the only cause of someone falling.

◆ It usually only part of a wider set of problems.

◆ The right footwear should hold the foot firmly, and provide as wide and solid a base as possible.

◆ The right shoe for someone with walking difficulties is not likely to be a fashion item, and may be difficult to buy in the local shops.

We wear something on our feet most of the time—slippers at home and shoes outside. Of all of the external things that can contribute to falls, footwear is with us the longest—most of the waking day—and therefore has the greatest opportunity to play some part when a crisis arises, and contribute to turning a stumble or trip into a fall.

Research has shown that falls are associated with certain types of footwear. In some studies, it is said that in up to a half of falls the footwear worn at the time was unsuitable, and may have contributed to the fall.

Footwear also plays a part when we are walking on uneven ground, or up stairs or kerbsides. At such times it is important that the footwear holds the foot snugly and does not move its position on the foot, leading to a sudden slip that would move the body's centre of gravity and cause a loss of balance.

What is the right sort of footwear?

The main points about footwear are:

◆ it should hold the foot firmly

◆ the heels should be not too high or too narrow

◆ the soles and heels should not be slippery

◆ shoes with laces hold the foot more firmly than slip-ons

◆ slippers should have support at the heel, rather than a sole that flops free at the back.

The evil of high heels!

High heels require better balance to stay upright. Usually they are also narrow, which reduces the available area for the body to balance on. The broader the heel, the easier it will be to retain balance when it is challenged.

High heels result in an abnormal posture, with abnormal positions of the ankles, hips, and lower back, impairing stability.

> Some women have worn high heels all their lives. Their muscles and tendons may have shortened and they find it very difficult or uncomfortable to walk on flat soles. In such cases a compromise needs to be found.

Buying the right kind of shoe is difficult enough when your feet are normal—not deformed, swollen, or painful. When you have feet that are affected by arthritis, bunions, or other conditions, it is very difficult to find anything that fits.

Swollen feet

A particular problem exists for those whose feet are swollen. This is a common problem that can have a number of causes. Often there has been damage to the vessels (called lymphatics) that drain the fluid from the leg. This is caused by infection, injury, surgery to the leg, or being overweight, or it may be an inherited tendency. Some people have had a previous injury to the leg, or a clot in the vein, which can cause persistent swelling. Others have swelling due to failure of the heart to pump strongly enough, although this can usually be controlled with water tablets.

Sandals with Velcro fastenings are the most suitable footwear, as they allow for the large changes in foot size that occur over the course of the day. Feet that are slim in the morning may be twice the size by the evening.

Buying the right shoes

The types of women's shoes that are available in the shops are dictated by fashion, rather than by comfort or safety. Many people find that mail order catalogues have a better selection of 'sensible shoes' than can be found in the high street. Advice about the right type of shoe for you can be obtained from a physiotherapist, who will usually know where they can be bought locally.

20

How can walking aids help?

→ Key points

◆ A walking stick gives the brain extra information about where the floor is and broadens the base of support to add stability.

◆ A Zimmer frame provides support and stability, but has to be lifted at every step.

◆ A wheeled Zimmer frame allows support, and is easier for walking.

◆ A delta frame has larger wheels and allows walking at a faster pace, but has limited stability.

◆ A trolley may contain a seat and a shopping bag.

Walking sticks

A walking stick is the most common aid that older people use to help with walking and balance. Some weight can be put through the stick, relieving the burden on a painful or stiff hip or knee joint to a minor extent. The amount of weight that can be transferred onto the stick is small, and a stick is not particularly good for this purpose as it is carried on one side and is not very comfortable to lean on. The walking stick effectively widens the area over which the body is stable.

A walking stick gives additional information about body position. Information from the hand holding the stick is much more sensitive than information from the legs.

151

The usefulness of a walking stick in gaining extra information can be shown easily. With the eyes shut, shaking the head from side to side does away with all visual and vestibular inputs. Balance is then entirely dependent on proprioception. This can be diminished further by standing on the toes. It is very hard to maintain such a position for more than a couple of seconds if the eyes are shut and the head is moving. However, when holding a walking stick, it becomes very much easier. The hand is very rich in nerve endings and these send information to a larger area in the brain than do the legs.

Many people are reluctant to be seen carrying a stick. Some use an alternative, such as a full-length umbrella, with which they feel more comfortable.

> Of all the things that happen in the falls clinic, the one thing that probably makes the greatest difference is educating people about walking aids, providing the most suitable aid for them, and encouraging them to use it.

How to assess the right length for a walking stick

Walking sticks need to be of the right length. This is assessed by standing up and letting the hand hang down by the side of the leg. The stick should reach from the floor, to the middle of the wrist. The stick should have a properly fitting non-stick (usually rubber) ferrule at the bottom.

The quadrupod (quad stick, four-footed stick)

A frame is not of any use for someone who is unable to use one arm—following stroke or a broken arm, for example. A walking stick gives limited support, but this can be increased by putting four small legs on the end of the stick, which is then called a quadrupod (Figure 20.1). This gives some sideways support.

> The riddle of the Sphinx, in the ancient Greek legend of Oedipus, asks: 'What creature walks on four legs, then two, then three, and then none.' The answer is man, who crawls as a baby before he can walk, then uses a stick, before being bedridden in old age. Clearly walking aids are not a new invention.

The Zimmer frame (frame without wheels)

A Zimmer frame has four legs spaced wide apart. It is robust and does not slip. It can take all of a patient's weight. It is useful for those who need a lot of

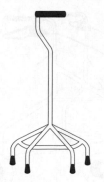

Figure 20.1 A quadrupod walking aid.

support and are unstable, particularly if their arms are strong. Its disadvantage is that, when walking, it needs to be picked up at every step. This breaks the natural rhythm of walking and gives a period of instability when there is no support. This means that it is only useful for those whose walking speed is very limited, and it is generally only used indoors.

The two-wheeled Zimmer frame (mobilator)

By putting wheels on the front two legs of the frame (Figure 20.2), the speed of walking can be increased, but at the cost of some stability. The frame can be moved forward without lifting, but it will not move when weight is put on it. It is more supportive than the frames described below, but needs to be lifted to make a turn. Narrow frames are available to fit through narrow doors at home.

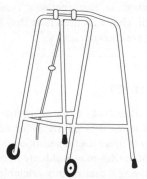

Figure 20.2 A wheeled Zimmer frame.

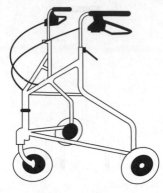

Figure 20.3 A delta frame.

The delta frame

For those who can walk at a reasonable pace, but who need some support at times, a delta frame is the best answer. This has one large wheel at the front and two side wheels, with the whole frame in a V shape (Figure 20.3). The handgrips have brakes, like those on a bicycle. Some have brakes that are activated when weight is put on the handgrips, so that it can be used by people whose grip strength is poor, such as those with severe arthritis of the hands.

Delta frames allow people to walk at a speed that is normal, or nearly so. They are manoeuvrable, but there is a risk of tipping over sideways when they are leant on with only one hand. The two sides fold together and therefore they take up less space in the house than other frames.

> For many people the stigma of 'being geriatric', and using an aid, is more than they can cope with. They wait until have they have fallen and broken something before they are convinced.

Four-wheeled frames

Four-wheeled frames (Figure 20.4) allow an uninterrupted gait, but do not allow much weight to be taken through them for support. Some have shopping baskets and a variety of other useful additions. Many have a shelf that can be used as a seat. For those who may suddenly need to sit down when they walk out of the house, having a seat readily available is a great advantage. In the house this seat can be used to carry things when both arms are needed to

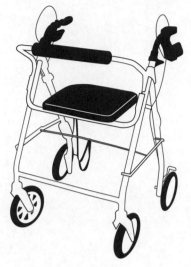

Figure 20.4 A four-wheeled trolley with seat.

use the trolley as a walking frame. A plate or other things can be put on the seat, and transported on the trolley.

- Zimmer frames are mostly for use in the home. Walking speeds are limited, and the small wheels of mobilators do not move easily over rough surfaces.

- Delta frames and four-wheeled frames have larger wheels, and can be used at greater speeds, making them useful outside the home.

21

What role do diet and vitamin deficiencies have in causing falls?

➔ Key points

A poor diet in the elderly is caused by:

- reluctance to cook

- lack of knowledge and experience in cooking (especially men)

- lack of hunger

- loss of 'taste' (in fact a loss of smell)

- difficulty doing the shopping

- being housebound

- poverty.

Nearly all older people are deficient in vitamin D.

Vitamin D supplements are the main treatment for osteoporosis, and should be given to anyone at risk of osteoporosis.

Vitamin B_{12} deficiency is not uncommon and can cause orthostatic hypotension (which may be reversible).

Poor diet and weight loss

Older people tend to have poor diets, and this has an adverse effect on their health. There are a number of reasons for this. In the popular press, poverty is put forward as a major reason, but this is probably not an important factor for the majority of older people.

Older men who become widowed may never have cooked for themselves, and may not be used to having to prepare their own food. Older women may always have cooked for someone else. They may not have particularly enjoyed cooking, and often cannot be bothered to cook for themselves.

A second factor is that some people stop feeling hungry, and they feed themselves only because they know that they have to. Some people lose their sense of smell as they grow older. The taste of food depends on the sense of smell, not taste (which distinguishes only sweet, sour, salty, and bitter, and does not tell you the taste of food). This loss of the sense of smell is a particular feature of dementias.

In addition, as people have increasingly limited mobility, it becomes more difficult for them to obtain fresh food. They tend to go shopping less often, or arrange for someone else to do it for them, and buy a limited range, often of prepared foods. Fresh fruit and vegetables may be a smaller part of their diet than it was when they did their own shopping. Carrying the shopping home may be a major obstacle.

> A large proportion of the elderly population is malnourished and they lose weight.
>
> The loss of muscle leads to decreased strength and hence a tendency to fall.
>
> In extreme cases the under-nutrition can be sufficient to cause loss of memory, fatigue, lassitude, and an inability to manage at home.

In some cases the diminished appetite is the result of an illness, such as cancer, peptic ulceration, or, very commonly, inflammation of the stomach caused by aspirin or painkillers. Generalized weight loss leads to weakness of the legs, and is a major cause of falls.

Vitamin deficiencies

Two particular vitamin deficiencies play an important role. These are deficiencies of vitamin D and vitamin B_{12}.

Vitamin D

Vitamin D deficiency is very common; most older people, and a large proportion of young people are vitamin D deficient. This deficiency is believed to be one of the main causes of osteoporosis—the thinning of the bones that makes older people so susceptible to fractures. It is also believed to play a part in maintaining muscle strength.

Most vitamin D is produced in the skin under the influence of sunlight. Vitamin D is found in oily fish, liver, and eggs. A variety of foods such as margarine, breakfast cereals, and bread are fortified with vitamin D. Even healthy adults tend to become deficient in vitamin D in the winter. Those with kidney disease, or who have little exposure to sunlight, are particularly prone to vitamin D deficiency.

Vitamin D supplements

Most older women would probably benefit from a vitamin D supplement, which is taken as a tablet. Usually this is combined with calcium supplements, and this mixture is available in a variety of preparations.

Calcium (1 gram) and vitamin D (800 units) tablets are the mainstay of treatment of osteoporosis. Everyone who has osteoporosis, or who is at risk of osteoporosis, should take this unless there is some medical reason not to do so (which is rare). Giving calcium and vitamin D has a beneficial effect on the skeleton. It is believed to have a beneficial effect on other body systems, although this is less well established.

How safe are vitamin D supplements?

For most people, calcium and vitamin D supplements are safe if taken in normal doses. As long as blood tests are done to check that there is no evidence of kidney failure and that the level of calcium in the blood is normal, it is very improbable that normal doses of calcium and vitamin D can do any harm.

Vitamin B_{12}

The body does not need a great deal of vitamin B_{12}, and usually has enough stored to last for many months. The problem arises when it ceases to be absorbed properly. One cause of poor absorption is pernicious anaemia, in which the body starts to produce an antibody (a type of protein) that affects the stomach lining in such a way that it ceases to produce intrinsic factor (IF). Vitamin B_{12} has to bind to IF in order to be absorbed.

Vitamin B_{12} deficiency is more common than is generally appreciated, but only a few of these people have pernicious anaemia. The cause in most people is not well understood, but there seems to be a problem with absorption over a prolonged period, often combined with a diet poor in vitamin B_{12}. There is some debate about what is a normal level of vitamin B_{12}, and difficulty with measuring it accurately at lower levels, but some authors estimate that one in seven older people has vitamin B_{12} deficiency.

> Vitamin B_{12} is found in red meat, and in smaller amounts in other foods, such as fish, dairy products, eggs, and yeast extracts. Many older people eat a predominantly chicken and fish diet, and get little vitamin B_{12} in their diet.

From the point of view of a falls clinic, vitamin B_{12} deficiency is important. It is the only curable cause of orthostatic hypotension (if we exclude stopping medications). It causes damage to the nerves that supply blood vessels so that they cannot respond to a change in posture to maintain the blood pressure. This may improve over a few months once vitamin B_{12} injections have been started.

> ## ✖ Myth
>
> 'Only people with anaemia have significant vitamin B_{12} deficiency.'
>
> Vitamin B_{12} is required for the function of two different enzyme systems, one in the bone marrow and one in the nervous system. Most patients with neurological symptoms never develop anaemia.

Vitamin B_{12} deficiency causes several other problems. It affects the peripheral nerves, causing numbness and tingling of the hands and feet. In severe cases, it can affect the spinal cord, and cause severe unsteadiness and weakness. It causes anaemia, but by a different mechanism to that affecting the nerves. Whether it can lead to a deterioration in memory or to dementia is unclear.

It is usually treated by regular injections of the vitamin every 3 months for life. More recently it has been found that large doses of the vitamin (1000 micrograms) in tablet form are a suitable treatment—if enough is given, an adequate amount is absorbed.

22

What causes falls in care homes?

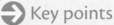 Key points

Care home residents have the greatest risk of falling of anyone in the population. Falling at home is the main reason that people go into care homes.

The risk of falling is highest in the first 2 weeks, and then steadily reduces.

Falls prevention in care homes involves:

- training the staff about falls

- assessing the patient's falls risk factors (especially medications)

- appropriate care plans

- use of alarms when appropriate

- eternal vigilance!

Falls are very common in care homes. In addition, most people in care homes are confused to a greater or lesser extent. Care homes contain two groups of people—those who can get up and walk (however unsafely), and those who cannot. Those who are unable to get out of their bed or chair without help are at low risk of falling (other than out of their bed or chair, or when being transferred). It is the other group, who are mobile but unsafe and who usually have some degree of confusion, who are the people at the highest risk of falling in the whole population.

Residential homes contain a small percentage of the elderly population, but account for 20 per cent of all patients admitted to hospital with a fractured hip.

The main reason that people give up their own homes to go into a care home is that they have had falls at home, or that they or their families fear that they might. This is usually combined with a degree of confusion or dementia, such that they are unable to manage themselves safely at home or to cope when they do fall. In a care home the patient is still likely to fall, but if they do, at least there will be someone there to help them.

When people move into a care home, they find themselves in a new environment, and it is in the first few weeks that they are at their greatest risk of falling. As they accustom themselves to their surroundings, and as the staff get to know them, the risk reduces. Often people who are confused become agitated in their new environment and do not always realize that there is someone around to help. They persist in trying to get up on their own.

Looking after people who fall in care homes is an enormous problem for those who manage them. Some falls are inevitable. The only way to prevent falls completely is to prevent people from moving around. Some risk has to be accepted, but every effort should be made to minimize it.

Care home staff need to be trained in how to maintain safety for this population. Such staff typically have a high rate of turnover, so that there are continually new and untrained members of staff working in care homes. Many of these are from other countries, and language may be a problem, in terms of both training and communicating with the patient. They have to come to understand the importance of falls, and must be motivated to do something about it. Often they will not understand that falls are largely preventable.

A major cause for falls in care homes is the amount of medication that patients receive. Commonly such patients will have confusion and agitation, and take regular sedatives or sleeping tablets. Many will be on antidepressants. A large number will be on treatments for high blood pressure and heart failure. All of these taken together are likely to make a great contribution to the risk of falling in someone who is confused and frail, and has poor mobility.

Occasionally there are individual patients who fall again and again. It is important that they are flagged up to the staff and the family as recurrent fallers, and that everything possible is done to prevent their falls before fractures render them completely immobile. They need to have:

◆   their medications reviewed

◆   a review of their walking aids

◆   their urine tested in case they have a urine infection

◆ a sensible review of how their room is organized (the heights of beds and chairs)

◆ an appropriate nursing care plan written for them (see Chapter 23).

Sometimes such patients will have been given the wrong walking aid, or that aid will be used wrongly. Often in care homes patients' walking aids have not been reviewed as their condition changes, and their frames or walking sticks may be inappropriate or in a poor condition. For example, the rubber ferrule at the end of the walking stick might have worn through, or the brakes on their wheeled frame may not work.

Hip protectors are of dubious value in preventing fractures, but what they do is to flag up the fact that the patient is a faller to the care staff, and thereby have a positive effect on the staff's treatment of that individual.

A major problem in care homes is that anxiety about falls causes the staff to discourage or limit the patient's walking. This is a difficult problem, as encouraging walking requires a lot of staff time and involves taking a risk. Often the patients themselves wants to be left alone to sit in a chair, and the ability to walk is lost.

> Whereas 50 per cent of people over 80 years of age fall each year, the rate of falling in care homes is much higher, with one study finding as many as 2.7 falls per resident per year on average. Typically a care home will have a large number of patients who fall rarely, if ever, a small number who fall fairly often, and one or two who are falling all the time. It is this last group that is the cause of such dramatic statistics.

Alarm systems which tell staff when someone has got up are effective. They work not by calling staff members, who are rarely close enough to respond fast enough to prevent a fall, but by training the patient to sit down when the alarm goes off. If the patient is sitting with others in a ward or a common room, other patients tell the patient to sit down in order to switch off the noise of the alarm. This leads to a modification of the patient's high-risk behaviour.

23

Why do people fall in hospital?

➲ Key points

◆ The risk factors for falls in hospital are well recognized.

◆ Risk assessment tools and appropriate care plans, and dealing with modifiable risk factors are the accepted approach.

◆ Bed rails (cot sides) are useful in the right cases.

◆ Formal risk assessment scores have been disappointing in their usefulness in different clinical settings.

Hospitals are supposed to be places of safety. People in hospital are looked after by nurses, whose first duty is to ensure their safety. It is difficult for patients and their families to accept that falls occur in hospital but, despite taking all the precautions we can, some falls cannot be prevented.

About a third of these falls result in a significant injury—usually bruising or a laceration. Fractures occur in about one in 50 cases, and head injuries are less common but may be serious.

There are well-recognized risk factors for falls in hospital:

◆ previous falls

◆ difficulty walking

◆ leg weakness

◆ confusion with agitation

◆ impaired judgement

◆ sedative medication

◆ urinary problems

   ◆ frequency

   ◆ urgency

   ◆ needing help when using the toilet.

Physical injury is only one of the consequences—loss of confidence, anxiety, and a backward step in recovery lead to a prolongation of the stay in hospital. Those who fall in hospital are less likely to return to their own homes.

❓ Where do patients fall when in hospital?

◆ 24% occurred while walking.

◆ 23% fell from bed.

◆ 14% fell from the toilet or commode.

◆ 11% fell from trolleys.

◆ 5% fell from chairs.

◆ 3% fell in bathrooms.

Most patients who fall are found near their beds or chairs. Those people who are fit enough to walk further are less likely to fall.

The fall causes anxiety and guilt for the patient's family, and also for hospital staff. There is often an assumption that something could have been done to prevent the fall, and that someone should be held to account for it. Falls in hospital often lead to litigation.

📄 Case history

Edna was an 84-year-old woman who lived alone and was independent. She had a knee replacement, and in the weeks after coming home from hospital started to be confused and disorientated for the first time in her life.

Her daughter brought her to stay with her, and her GP took some blood, which showed a very low level of sodium. She was sent to hospital.

In hospital, her low sodium was treated, but she remained confused and agitated. She was fully mobile, and while walking around the ward, she toppled over and fell, hitting her head. She did not sustain any significant injury, but greater care was taken in keeping an eye on her.

Two days later she went to bed in the evening, and bed rails were put up at the side of her bed to prevent her from falling out of bed. She slid herself down the bed, and climbed out of the end, falling on the floor as she did so.

This time she broke her hip. She required an operation to repair it. After the operation she was very muddled, but things settled after a few days.

She spent many months in hospital recovering from her fracture. She had several infections and developed pulmonary emboli (clots in the lung), a potentially fatal complication.

Both of her falls occurred within a few feet of one of the nursing staff. On both occasions the nurse was just a little too far away to prevent her falling.

I subsequently reviewed her case in detail with her family, and it was clear that every possible precaution had been taken to minimize the chance of her falling, but despite our best efforts, she had two falls in hospital, resulting in an operation and a prolonged illness. In retrospect, she had probably had a small stroke (later confirmed on a brain scan) at the time of her knee operation which caused her confusion and agitation.

Some patients will be at risk of falling throughout their hospital stay because of a combination of risk factors. For others, there is a period of high risk during the initial stages of their treatment, which diminishes over time as their health improves, they become stronger and steadier on their feet, and they become used to their surroundings and perhaps less muddled. About half of inpatient falls occur in the first 10 days in hospital.

Only 4–5 per cent of falls are witnessed by staff. Even when a staff member is with the patient as they fall, they may not be able to prevent it. It is not possible to hold up someone whose legs have given way under them, and usually the most that can be hoped for is that the fall will be more gentle and less likely to result in injury.

If someone is immobile, getting them back on their feet involves a stage in which they are at great risk of falling. They are able to do things, but not to do them safely, and have to be left to get on with it in order to make progress.

What can be done to prevent falls in hospital?

Obviously the main step in preventing falls is to get the patient as well and as strong as they possibly can be. In addition, nurses' awareness that the patient might fall needs to be raised, so that the right steps are taken to make things safe for them.

Preventing falls in hospital may involve several stages:

◆ assessment of whether the patient has risk factors

◆ a falls risk score

◆ a nursing care plan

◆ information on falls for patients and their families.

This can be done in several ways, and which one is used depends upon the circumstances.

◆ Who is being looked after?

◆ Are they are in hospital, a care home, or somewhere else?

What is important is that these assessments should lead to actions being taken to reduce the risk of falls. Rather than just fill in pieces of paper that predict falls, we should do things to prevent falls.

One important study looked at modifiable risk factors, rather than risk assessments:

◆ diagnosing the cause of delirium

◆ reducing sedative medications

◆ diagnosing and treating infections

◆ checking lying and standing blood pressure

◆ checking vision

◆ ensuring that the right walking aids are available.

Bed rails (cot sides)

Protective side rails, which limit the chances of the patient falling out of bed, can be attached to the sides of hospital beds. These used to be called 'cot sides', but this term implies the return of the older person to the status of an infant and is now seen as unacceptable. Many staff are reluctant to use them—those used in the past often had sharp edges, and led to injuries. Some staff see them as a form of restraint and an infringement of the patient's liberty, but research with patients and their families shows that their use is accepted and even welcomed by most people.

They are useful in selected cases. They may prevent someone from falling out of bed or from trying to climb out of bed when muddled or disorientated. However, for some patients who are confused and agitated, they are not a barrier to getting out of bed. Commonly they slide down to the end of the bed, and try and climb out where the bed rails end. This often leads to falls and injuries.

On balance, bed rails lead to a reduction in injuries, particularly serious injuries to the head and the hip. An experienced nurse should be able to judge who will benefit from bed rails.

Bed rail assessment

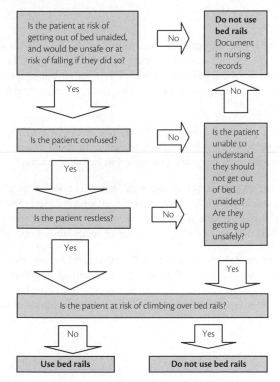

The need for bed rails should be reviewed at least twice a week, or after any falls.

◆ Ensure that bed rails are aligned against the side of the mattress to minimize the risk of entrapment.

◆ Where bed rails are used, either nurse the patient close to the nurses' station, or institute hourly observations to reduce the likelihood of the patient being trapped between the rails.

◆ If the patient is restless, ensure that padded bed rails are available to reduce the risk of injury.

◆ Decisions to use or to stop using bed rails, and the reasons for them, must be documented in the nursing records.

📋 Case history

John was an 81-year-old man who was found on the floor by his wife. He had slurred speech and was not moving his left arm and leg. He denied that there was anything wrong with him. When an ambulance was called, he refused to go to hospital and needed an hour of persuasion before he would agree.

He could not see to his left side, and was not aware of anything on that side (a hemianopia with sensory neglect). He continued to deny that anything was wrong with him, and demanded to be taken home.

He kept trying to get out of bed, but was unable to take his weight on his left leg and would have fallen if not restrained. Bed rails were put up, and he was not physically able to get out over them or to climb out over the end of the bed. He realized this, and stopped trying to get up.

By the following day his condition had settled, and he accepted that he was unable to get out of bed. The bed rails had helped to prevent an injury when he was disorientated. He wished to keep them now he was better, as they made him feel more secure and less likely to roll out of bed.

Examples of different forms of falls risk assessments and plans

A falls risk assessment

Gait

Do they have difficulty with their gait or balance?

If yes:

Do they usually walk with a walking aid?

If not, or if they do not have their aid with them, or if it is the wrong aid:

Refer to physiotherapy.

If they remain unsteady:

Ensure supervision during transfers and walking.

Agitation

Are they agitated or confused, or do they have cognitive impairment?

Is this normal for them? If not:

Consider an underlying cause:

infection: check temperature, respiratory rate, pulse, blood pressure, test urine;

medication, especially anything new, analgesics, sedatives.

Consider:

Do they wander?

Do they need close observation?

Is the environment free from hazards?

Are they wearing their glasses?

Is their footwear appropriate?

History of falls

Do they have a history of falls?

Has the cause of the previous falls been identified?

If not discuss with the medical team.

Blood pressure

Are they taking any medication that will affect their pulse or blood pressure?

Is the systolic blood pressure below 110 mmHg?

Measure the blood pressure lying down and then standing up using a manual sphygmomanometer. If the systolic blood pressure drops by 20 mmHg or more, inform the medical team.

Medication

Are they taking any medication for high blood pressure or heart disease that might reduce the blood pressure excessively?

Are they taking antidepressants or sedatives?

Continence

Are they incontinent of urine? Do they have urinary frequency?

If so:

Position the patient close to a toilet and offer frequent assistance with toileting.

Do they have a urine infection?

Ensure that their call bell is within reach at all times.

Following an assessment using the above 'triggers', please complete an individual care plan that documents the patient's risk of falling and what interventions are planned.

Sensory impairment

Do they need glasses or hearing aids, and are these in good condition, and within reach?

Falls care plan (based on the York trial)

History of falls before admission	Yes/No
Fall since admission	Yes/No
Tries to walk alone but unsteady/unsafe	Yes/No
Patient or relatives anxious about falls	Yes/No
If yes to any of the questions above, complete the care plan	Actions taken

Goal: to reduce the likelihood of falls whilst maintaining dignity and independence.

Call bell: Ensure that the call bell has been explained and is in reach. Consider alternatives for those unable to use the call bell, such as moving the patient nearer the nurses' station.

Eyesight: Ensure that eyesight has been checked.

Check that glasses are available and suitable, if worn.

Is the patient (wearing glasses, if needed) able to identify a pen or key from a bed length away?

Request medical review of eyesight if the patient is unable to see objects as above.

Bed and bed rails: Assess the need for bed rails.

If likely to fall from bed, ensure that the bed is at the lowest possible height, unless this would reduce mobility or independence. Consider the use of a special low bed.

Medication: Check for medication associated with falls risk, e.g. antidepressants, sedatives, anti-psychotics. Ask doctor to review. Do not stop abruptly.

Multi-disciplinary team: Ensure that members of the team are aware of falls risk, and are taking appropriate action according to their protocols and clinical need.

Footwear: Check footwear for secure fit, non-slip sole, no trailing laces. Arrange safer replacement from family or ward store. Consider slipper socks in bed for patients at risk of falling at night.

Place: Nurse in the most appropriate place on the wards for their needs—close to nurses' station, toilet, or somewhere quiet (taking other patients' needs into account).

Lighting: Consider lighting that is best for the patient—bedside lamp left on or nightlight in toilet.

Urinalysis: Perform urinalysis. Send midstream urine if positive for blood, nitrates, or protein.

Toilet: Does the risk of falls appear to be associated with the patient's need to use the toilet?

If so, a routine of frequent toilet visits may prevent falls.

Lying and standing blood pressure: Measure and record lying and standing blood pressure. If systolic drop is greater than 20 mmHg, inform the doctor. Advise patient on getting up slowly.

> **Inform**: Provide falls leaflet to patient and family. Engage them in care planning. Check contact wishes in case of fall.

Falls risk assessment scores

It was hoped that a scoring system would be able to highlight who was at risk of falling on the ward, so that action could be targeted at them to prevent falls. A score that works well in one area does not seem to work as well in a different hospital, or on a different type of ward. There is a great temptation for busy staff to record the risk of falls, but then to do nothing about it. Such scores correctly identify a high percentage of patients on a ward as being at high risk of falling, but do not identify which one or two will actually fall.

The best known of these scores is STRATIFY. A number of risk factors for falls were tested, and the contribution they made to the risk of falls was calculated. The five that predicted falls best were incorporated into a scoring system which was validated in another hospital. Despite this scientific approach, STRATIFY has not fulfilled expectations.

> ## Stratify
>
> Did the patient present to hospital with a fall, or has the patient fallen while in hospital?
>
> Yes = 1 No = 0
>
> Do you think the patient is agitated?
>
> Yes = 1 No = 0
>
> Do you think the patient is visually impaired to the extent that visual function is affected?
>
> Yes = 1 No = 0
>
> Do you think the patient is in need of especially frequent toileting?
>
> Yes = 1 No = 0
>
> Does the patient have a high transfer and mobility score?
>
> Yes = 1 No = 0
>
> A score of 2 or more predicted falling in the next week with a sensitivity of 93 per cent and a specificity of 88 per cent in the local validation study.

24

What should I do if I fall?

➡️ Key points

If you fall and are unable to get up:

- summon help
- move to a soft surface
- keep moving
- keep warm
- try to get off the floor.

Make sure you wear your pendant alarm at all times, and use it when you fall to summon help.

If you fall over, you will probably feel a little shocked or shaken. Take some slow deep breaths, try to stay calm, and plan what action to take.

If you are hurt or unable to get up

- **Try to summon help:**

  - use your pendant alarm if you have one

  - bang on the wall or floor to get your neighbour's attention

  - call out for help

  - crawl or shuffle on your bottom towards the phone, dial 999 and ask for an ambulance, or call a neighbour, relative, or friend.

- **Move to a soft surface** if you are able to. If you have fallen on a hard floor, try to move to a carpeted area away from draughts.

◆ **Keep moving** Do not lie in one position for too long as you may become cold or develop pressure areas. If you can, roll from side to side from time to time, or change your position, or regularly tense your arms and legs.

◆ **Keep warm** Reach for something nearby to cover yourself, such as a blanket, coat, or tablecloth (as long as it will not bring heavy objects onto you). You might find it helpful to keep a small blanket in a low cupboard or tucked away behind some furniture in each room. A bottle of water might also help prevent dehydration if you have to lie for a long time.

If you have to empty your bladder, find something to soak it up and move away from the wet area.

If you are unhurt, try to get up

Roll over onto your hands and knees. If you have difficulty turning from your back onto your side, the following sequence of movements may help (Figure 24.1).

◆ Bend your knees and let them drop to the side you are turning to.

◆ Turn your head in the direction of the roll.

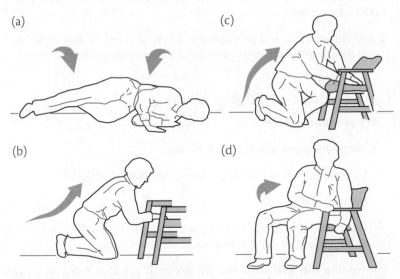

(a)

(b)

(c)

(d)

Figure 24.1 Getting up from the floor.

◆ Reach over with your uppermost arm.

◆ Crawl to a stable piece of furniture such as a bed, stool, or chair without castors. Approach from the front and put both hands on the seat.

◆ With your hands on the support, place the foot of your stronger leg on the floor. Lean forwards and push yourself up (rocking and counting may help).

◆ As you rise, twist round and sit on the seat. Rest for a while before getting up.

Tell your doctor you have had a fall, even if you are unhurt, as you may need advice or treatment to help prevent further falls.

'The long lie'

One of the problems that is most feared by patients and staff is being unable to get up or to summon help, and finding yourself on the floor for many hours, or even days. This is termed 'the long lie'. Any fall where the patient is on the floor for more than an hour is deemed to be a long lie.

Four out of five falls happen when the patient is on their own. In about one in five falls, there is a long lie. There are many factors that may contribute to being unable to get up, the most obvious being an injury. The only factor that is found consistently is confusion or dementia. The risk in someone with dementia of a fall resulting in a long lie is about six times greater than for someone who is not forgetful.

Many patients have a pendant alarm, but do not wear it. A typical comment is: 'I don't have to wear my pendant yet'. Some people are flustered or forgetful, and cannot remember that they have it. Others do not want to use it because they do not want to disturb the person who would be summoned to help them.

For some people, not calling for help is about trying to maintain their autonomy. For others, it is a fear of being taken to hospital and never coming back. Some people who fall outside think that the alarm will not work in the garden, and do not use it.

Sheltered housing complexes have pull cords in every room, which usually go right down to the floor so that they can be activated by someone lying on the ground. These can be a hazard in themselves, in that people are afraid to turn the lights on in the bathroom for fear of pulling the alarm cord—something that most of us who work in hospital will have done at some stage. Not having lights on in the bathroom and the transition from a well-lit living room to a dark bathroom present a significant falls risk.

Hypothermia

Lying on the floor, even on the carpet of a warm centrally heated room, is a significant cold stress. Heat is lost to the floor, and a small percentage of susceptible individuals may develop hypothermia. It is important to keep warm and to keep moving if you do find yourself on the floor.

Glossary

Acoustic neuroma A growth on the nerve leading from the ear, which can cause deafness and vertigo. It is not cancerous, and can be removed surgically. It is diagnosed by an MRI scan of the brain.

Atrial fibrillation An irregular chaotic pulse rhythm. Going into atrial fibrillation from a normal (sinus) rhythm causes a sudden drop in blood pressure, which can result in a variety of symptoms. Some people are persistently in atrial fibrillation, but may have moments when the heart speeds up so that it does not have sufficient time to fill up in each beat, reducing the amount it can pump. Atrial fibrillation may lead to clots forming in the heart, which can cause strokes.

Autonomic neuropathy A condition in which nerves supplying blood vessels, the gut, and some other organs deteriorate. It can cause problems with blood pressure, most commonly orthostatic hypotension.

Balance: dynamic The ability to remain balanced while moving.

Balance: static The ability to remain balanced while standing.

Base of support The area above which we are standing, corresponding to a line drawn around our feet and any other object providing support (such as a walking stick).

Benign positional vertigo A common condition affecting the inner ear. Small pieces of chalk become displaced and enter the semicircular canals, giving rise to false information on movement. This causes vertigo on certain head movements. It is treated by Epley's manoeuvre.

Brainstem The area where nerve fibres from various parts of the brain come together to enter the spinal cord in order to reach the rest of the body, and in which some vital nerves have their origins (called nerve nuclei). Damage to this small area can have a disproportionate effect, as so many different nerves are packed together very tightly.

Carotid sinus hypersensitivity A poorly understood condition in which there appears to be an over-sensitivity of nerves in a part of the carotid artery called the carotid sinus. These nerves are involved in the control of pulse and blood pressure. When over-sensitive, they cause sudden drops in the blood pressure or periods in which the heart stops beating for a few seconds.

Cataract Thickening of the lens of the eye, so that it does not let light through normally. A simple operation is required to remove the cataract and restore normal sight.

Cerebellum The back part of the brain, concerned with the control of movement and balance.

Contrast sensitivity The ability to distinguish one object from the next, particularly if they are similar in colour. Important on stairs where it is needed to tell where one step finishes and the next begins.

Delirium A deterioration in memory and understanding caused by some illness. It often leads to agitation and confusion. It is reversible.

Dementia An illness in which the brain cannot process thoughts properly. The loss of memory for recent events is the most noticeable symptom. It is not reversible, but treatments may slow the progression of the disease in some cases.

Depth perception The ability to determine where one object is placed in relation to another.

DEXA scan An X-ray scan used to measure the density of bone to diagnose osteoporosis. It stands for dual energy X-ray absorptiometry.

Drugs The terms 'drugs' and 'medicines' are used completely interchangeably by doctors, and the term does not imply illicit substances.

Foot drop A condition in which the muscles that raise the foot up are paralysed. It is seen following a stroke, or when nerves are trapped leaving the spinal column, or when the nerve to these muscles is damaged just below the knee.

Glaucoma A condition in which the pressure of fluid in the eye is raised. This can happen suddenly (acute glaucoma), when the eye becomes red and painful, or more slowly. The slow form is common and leads to a gradual loss of vision due to compression of the blood vessels to the nerves in the eye, causing them to die off.

Hemianopia Vision to one side of the body is lost in both eyes, most commonly following a stroke. Things on that side (and possibly almost straight ahead) are not in the patient's field of vision.

Hypertension High blood pressure.

Intrinsic and extrinsic factors for falls Intrinsic factors are those within the person themselves—arthritis, stroke, muscle weakness, poor balance, etc. Extrinsic factors are those in the person's surroundings—a wet floor, inappropriate footwear, etc.

Limits of stability An imaginary area around the body. When the centre of gravity is moved outside this area, balance cannot be maintained without some adjustment, usually by taking a step.

Macular degeneration Dying back of nerves in the middle of the retina, at the back of the eye. These are the nerves that supply the area that is being looked at—the middle part of the visual field. It makes reading and everyday activities difficult.

Ménière's disease A condition affecting the inner ear leading to vertigo, deafness, and ringing in the ears (tinnitus).

Orthostatic hypotension A drop in blood pressure on standing up.

Osteoporosis A thinning of the bones, leading to an increased chance of fractures.

Parkinson's disease A disease resulting in shaking, stiffness, and slow movements. Patients with Parkinson's disease are very prone to falling for a number of different reasons.

Peripheral neuropathy A deterioration of the nerve supply to the arms and legs. It may cause numbness, coldness, or tingling of the feet, or simply loss of balance. There are many causes, but usually no specific cause is found.

Postural giddiness Giddiness on movement. Most commonly this is on standing up, but can occur on lying flat, or with any other head movement.

Proprioception Body sensation. The sensation that comes from nerves in the skin, muscles, joints, and tendons telling the brain where it is in space.

Seizures, fits, and epilepsy 'Seizures' is the correct medical term for epileptic fits. Epilepsy is the disease characterized by recurrent seizures.

Sensory inattention and neglect Sensory neglect is a lack of awareness of one part of the body. Most commonly this is seen after a stroke, when the patient is unaware of one side of the body and often of anything going to that side. It is commonly accompanied by a hemianopia (see above). Sensory inattention is a milder version of sensory neglect. The patient is aware of things to the affected side, as long as there are not too many other stimuli drowning out that information. When attention is drawn to things on the normal side, the awareness of what is happening on the affected side decreases.

Small vessel disease Tiny areas of stroke within the deep brain substance which have a cumulative effect.

Stereoscopic vision The ability to see things with both eyes, and to use this information to judge distance.

Stroke A loss of brain function caused by the blockage of a blood vessel in the brain or by bleeding within the brain.

Supraventricular tachycardia A very rapid regular heart beat. This gives rise to an awareness of the heart beat (palpitations) and can cause a reduction in blood flow to the brain.

Syncope Loss of consciousness because of an inadequate blood supply to the brain. Giddiness due to a drop in blood supply to the brain is termed pre-syncope.

Transient ischaemic attack (TIA) A mini-stroke, in which the symptoms (but not necessarily the damage to the brain) have resolved within 24 hours. It is often the herald of a stroke in the following days, and needs urgent investigation and treatment to diminish the chances of a larger stroke.

Vasovagal syndrome, fainting A drop in blood pressure, often with warning symptoms of giddiness beforehand, sweating, and visual changes.

Vestibular neuronitis A viral infection affecting the nerves to the inner ear, causing vertigo that may last for many weeks. In some cases the nerves suffer some permanent damage, resulting in long-term unsteadiness.

Vestibular system The mechanism of the inner ear that tells us where we are in space.

Visual acuity The ability to see the objects you are looking at clearly.

Index